BIODYNAMICS OF OSTEOPATHY

Phase Four

Second Edition

James Jealous D.O.

For more information about Dr. Jealous please visit:
https://BiodynamicsOfOsteopathy.com

BIODYNAMICS OF OSTEOPATHY Phase Four

Hardback ISBN: 979-8-2955-3925-1

Second Edition 2025

James Jealous D.O. (1943–2021) practiced as an osteopathic physician, teacher and writer for many years. His life's work was to found and develop the specific methodology of Biodynamics of Osteopathy, following the lineage of Dr. A.T. Still and Dr. W.G. Sutherland.

This is one of a series of Biodynamics of Osteopathy books. They grew organically from sets of handouts written by Dr. Jealous and given to students during courses taught by him and his teachers. After many years he collected the handouts together and created individual course manuals, which he added to and rewrote many times. After several more years they evolved further into books.

TABLE OF CONTENTS

OSTEOPATHY IS SERVICE

We use our hands ...

To treat the Whole patient

To listen to the indwelling movements of Life

To treat all levels of illness

To assist in building the patient's functional reserve

To support homeostasis and trophicity by balancing the activity of the autonomic nervous system

To explore "laws not framed by human hands" (Dr. Still and Dr. Sutherland)

To cooperate and communicate with the Laws of Nature (Dr. Wales)

"To find the Health" (Dr. Still)

To get to the treatment plan

To get to the diagnosis

To help establish a point of Rest or Neutral around which the Whole can come to balance

To find Cause

We believe ...

We have an innate capacity to heal

The patient functions as a whole

The autonomic nervous system plays a major role in disease and healing

Structure and function are one form of activity

The Divine is indwelling

Life moves beyond death

There is a Constant Movement toward Normal

We are here to Serve Humanity

Normal is ...

"A sense of peace and harmony" (Dr. Sutherland)

Ease of motion, without tension

A capacity for Neutral

A sense of Wholeness to Life

The capacity for adaptation, change without compensation.

"Skill is proportionate to one's understanding of normal" (Dr. Still)

REVIEW: PHASES ONE THROUGH THREE

Phase One highlights "the Health."

We synchronize with the Health before we do anything else with the patient (see page 36 of the 1953 *OCA Journal*).

We worked with "motion present" in the lesion. This requires no motion testing. We followed local and systemic neutrals.

We began to discriminate between the various rates.

Stillpoints, Pauses, and Neutral were explored through their differences.

Our work in Phase Two focused not only on Synchronization with the Breathing of Primary Respiration but also added the skill of "Sensing the Fulcrum"; i.e., the Stillness around and through which the Breathing is creating its pattern and rate.

We began our study of the Fluid Body, accepting the difficult task of discriminating Zone A and Zone B.

"Automatic Shifting" was discovered to be diagnostic as well as therapeutic.

Phase Three moved our attention to the Sea Around Us, and the slower, softer, more patient breathing of the Long-Tide. We explored an Indwelling Therapeutic Force that was "waiting" to express its potency.

We saw how CV4 and EV4 were the same process, reestablishing Neutral in the Whole.

We studied the "Sacs."

Phase Four: We enter more deeply into the living Tide.

The Midline functions to center us in such a way that we become naturally aware of Zone D and the Dynamic Stillness in The Sea Around Us. This is not Zone A, Zone B, or the Long-Tide.

The Midline is not a line, but a place where the spatial relationships are expressed as a whole ... it is a function, not an anatomical structure.

The Midline is the sanctuary of the Health and its therapeutic forces.

PHASE FOUR LANGUAGE

The language developed here is for Biodynamics, to facilitate our need to communicate. Language only has meaning in the context of its history.

There is, regrettably, no such thing as objective language, except perhaps "The Voice of Silence."

The Dynamic Stillness

An Ocean of Serenity and Wisdom, no rates, only Stillness ... It is larger than Zone D.

The Midline

The river where the Whole originates and is centered for an individual. It is an Ocean of Creation.

The Sea Around Us

An Ocean of Diverse Life. It has many qualities and attributes.

"Life is the substance that fills all spaces of the Universe." (A. T. Still)

Transmutation of Consciousness

A shift in Perception that happens without your effort (except waiting) ... one is here ... a second later one is in a new landscape ... this is a key element for the rest of the Phases ... it changes all knowledge into a new category, the movement of the Wisdom of the Tide. The senses change from one state to another.

Ignition

The movement of The Potency of the Tide. Fire. The spark of Life. The power that drives the Engine of Life (words inherited from Still and Sutherland). A function of the Midline.

Deity

The Divine ... The Creator ... Love ... God

Third Level Stillness, The Dynamic Stillness

The stillness that centers us. One does not "go" to the Dynamic Stillness; one is carried there, blind ... often so quickly that one could think, "I did it."

Protoplasm

Usually seen as the first moldable substance that can hold an image.

Potency

Potency with a capital *P* denotes the absolute power of the movement and intention of the Breath of Life. Omnipotence. Holy Fire. Potency with a small *p* denotes relative potency that is generated to compensate for loss of response on our part to big *P*. This little potency is related to Rates, not the Dynamic Stillness. This little tide can be directed by one's will; the Big *P* cannot.

Transmutation

The conversion into something different. The conversion of one species into another species. A change in the whole.

Light

The soft radiance of the Health. The luminosity of uncreated light. This is not protonic light (sunlight). In newborns this is dramatic.

A wet sponge absorbs water more quickly than a dry one; let the Tide Center you.

"Life of the calm force, sent forth by Deity, to vivify all Nature" ... Dr. Still.

"Osteopathy is only in its infancy, it is an unknown sea, just discovered, and as yet, we are only acquainted with its shore tide." (Andrew Taylor Still, M.D., D.O., *Philosophy of Osteopathy*, Preface, 1899)

Space opens, then function moves in the Direction of Ease to express form.

"Slip along the breath into the Health" – St. Theresa

All the Zones begin at a Central Stillness and end in a Natural boundary.

Empty into the Emptiness

Find the Simple

Recommended reading:

"Be Still and Know," R. Becker, D.O., 1965 Sutherland Lecture

"Fulcrums," T. Schooley, D.O., 1953 *OCA Journal*

INTRODUCTION TO PHASE FOUR

The Midline is not a structure.

The word Midline has many levels of understanding and can be seen from many vantage points.

In Osteopathy there is no Midline ... The idea never entered the mainstream until the Biodynamic Model was proposed (1990) and accepted by many as they studied the application of the "Principles in Practice" of the Midline.

Osteopathy, as I was taught it and as the postgraduate courses presented it, never talked about a Midline ... the line of Gravity, certainly, but never an organizational force that provided the spatial dynamics of both growth and healing.

In 1990, I interviewed many experts, all of them Fellows of the American Academy of Osteopathy ... none used the idea and did not see Fryette as having presented a Fulcrum for his "Laws" ... some discussed the line of Gravity but none except Colin Dove, D.O., from England, could teach me how to palpate the relationship of the patient to the "Line."

Later, it became clear to me that Sutherland did see a Midline in the Fluid and also in the Extremities.

The Biodynamic Model of Primary Respiration has no absolute conclusion; it is open to birth or death.

As it appears today, in light of what we experience as a community of Traditional Osteopaths, and in light of what Science has to offer, one can appreciate several levels of understanding concerning the Midline, all of which are applicable to patient care.

The most concrete level is the Notochordal Midline ... the center of orientation for the Embryological Segments, and of the process of Synchronization for the unfolding of the Segments as a single movement ... Segmentation of the Embryo is a Neural, Visceral,

Somatic unfolding and is not related to the Vertebral Segments as seen in *Gray's Anatomy*. Looking at a vertebral segment as a Segment limits the therapeutic portals.

The Notochord is central to the true segments and extends from the tip of the coccyx to the junction of the Pre and Post Sphenoid, where its cranial end sits under the center of the diaphragm sellae and the lamina terminalis.

Laterally, from this cranial tip is the s-s pivot which Sutherland described so clearly. Anterior to the notochord in the cranium, the spatial orientation is to another Midline. Superiorly are the pituitary—the Ignition point for the Engine and Bregma.

My point is to make us think beyond the general facts and look deeper.

It seems possible that the Longitudinal Fluctuation, as described by Sutherland's students, is aligned to the notochord ... Remember, the Longitudinal Fluctuation only occurs at two to three cycles per minute, and the Notochordal Midline is definitely not related to the Long-Tide, so its importance is limited to specific arenas.

It is reabsorbed after segmentation is mature.

The Embryology texts discuss the Notochord Midline and usually intimate that it arises as an evolution of the Primitive Streak. But maybe there is something hidden from their instruments. I believe and sense another possible way of looking at this "primitive streak," and I will say more later.

The next Midline we speak about is the Line of Folding. This Midline is the Line to which, and from which, the form and geometry of the Seams occurs. This is covered in Phase Five. The foldings in the Whole Embryo occur everywhere and the Fulcrum is not in the notochord. The facial arches are a good example ... these folds are moving around a line of Orientation that is not the Notochord ... Another example would be the visceral movements of growth ... like the two halves of the uterus finding their final destination ... if one looks at the pictures in the texts one can see that there is a Midline, unseen by Embryologists but present for the spatially accurate movements and final position for and union of the sides of the uterus ... This Midline positions the parts with respect to the Whole ... when approached, this Midline creates Therapeutic Forces that clearly exchange with the Long-Tide, and if a Neutral occurs, another Midline is seen as Central to the Movement of Wholeness. Breathing of the Whole on the Long-Tide is related to this Midline that we attend during CV4 and EV4 application in the Direction of Ease.

The Movement of the Wholeness of the Incarnating Form, without any sense of the Parts, gives the impression of Spatial Dynamics that are Oriented to and Created from a Hollow Midline that is larger than the Soma ... Here a Dynamic Stillness flows into Creation not subjugated to any internal midline but capable of Creating them. This formlessness is informing from a Cause that appears to be Outside and through the Organism ... This Midline is the Midline for the Creation of the Whole as a Part of a greater Wholeness. This Midline is our connection with Cause, but we cannot just "go there" ... we must be carried by the Tide.

At each level the "substance" of the Midline is different.

We will follow these Principles as we travel along in the Courses ... Do not think about what I have said beyond the point where you have given way to Ignorance and the Freedom to explore, without restraining concepts ... From there you can remain empty and Neutral, a state that will allow you to find answers. These ideas are Living Realities.

The Mystery of the Midline is one of the Beauties of Creation ... As you will see, the True Midline will Center you rather than you going to it, which is futile and false.

The Midline Centers Us.

It Centers, Holds Us "On Its Center."

One "Becomes Wellness"

This Provides Us with a "Meeting Place," to Wait

For the Master

MEDITATION: "CENTERING AROUND THE EDGES"

Meditation is a word that brings to mind a variety of images and ideas.

The oldest use of meditation is that of a tool used to awaken oneself to other levels of being, to a realization that formatted thinking is not the only form of knowledge.

The tools used in meditation involve specific methods of mental activity such as chanting, posture, imaging, breathing, prayer, etc. Meditations are used to increase one's awareness of the Health and its activities.

The use of meditation throughout the history of humanity is proof of its necessity in developing awareness that goes beyond the common preoccupations of everyday life.

One example of the use of meditation is the chanting of the sutras in Yoga. The ancient Sanskrit is chanted to unlock the Memory of Eternity, to bring the heart into Wholeness. Repetition becomes a task that opens the understanding and actions of the disciple to a new Mind, capable of Freedom and Love.

In Christianity, one of the most famous meditations is the Rosary. For many, Mary represents the perfect Neutral, the selfless emptiness capable of knowing the Divine. The Rosary is very difficult. It requires chanting, sensing, and visualization of an episode in Christ's life all at once. This opens a door to a deeper sense of the Reality behind Christ's Presence.

All traditions have meditation, and study of the similarities is refreshing and very humbling.

Repetition and practice are at the core of any meditational format. The outcome is not perfecting the meditation, but rather establishing an inner reality that reaches beyond the self-centered mind and into a sensitivity of something Higher. The outcome cannot be known beforehand.

Once the meditation creates a new awareness, the awareness ripens by its own momentum. In other words, meditation awakens us to faculties that have been banished into the subconscious. These faculties are imprisoned by our social-educational-religious structures, by our egos, by our familial and genetic patterns, and by the natural tendency to "overthink" that has become the virus of civilization.

One could be overwhelmed by the resistance to reawakening these faculties except that the tendency toward Normal, toward Wholeness, toward Health, is so powerful that if we can come to Neutral through the discipline of meditation, we will be carried the rest of the way.

The doors of the prison open when we stop being held by old habits.

The power that supports, creates, heals, and Loves us (all of us) is waiting at the prison gate to allow the faculties to be free, to become the modus operandi of our sensorium. The Health will not force you to leave; you must choose, through concentration on the method you choose.

Meditation in the context of Osteopathic Thinking is a movement toward Neutral in oneself.

From this, one is slowly freed from mental shortcomings. This allows the attention to function easily in relationship to the more subtle and powerful activities of Primary Respiration.

Once the Tide is easily in our awareness, it centers, embraces, and nurtures us.

When the relationship with the Tide is established, the meditation is abandoned for the more direct activity of contemplation, which involves long periods of inner silence in the Presence of that which the Tide holds Sacred.

Meditation begins as an Active Effort, an act of will.

In Phase Four, we will actively center ourselves "around the edges." Why? To transform, holding our attention inside the place where all the worldly influences have placed it, our head, our self-centeredness, in the hope of projecting a false identity... The cave of aloneness.

We experience our "self" as having an identity as a person with certain attributes, most of which are only imaginary projections from the sources that have imprisoned the truer faculties, that are hidden from our awareness.

We will move our attention to "around the edges." Notice what happens to Zone A and Zone B with just this one step. How easy is it to stay outside and rest?

Watch ...

How often do you slip inside? And when you do, what happens to Zone A and Zone B? Moving oneself to a new location, like moving your home, is a big deal.

Sometimes you can think you are outside "around the edges" and you will be inside, thinking you are outside ... this is a projection ... something worth knowing.

The Method

1. Center around the edge of your skin, and feel the heat moving from the periphery.
2. Wait, watch the movement of your attention ... does it stay outside?
3. After a while you can sense another movement coming through the skin toward the periphery, as if you were transparent ... This is the Fluid Body RTP (reciprocal tension potency). Just watch ...
4. After a while, if you are outside and resting, the Fluid Body Tide creates a form.
5. Notice that your consciousness keeps slipping back inside ... Do not resist, just return to the outer edges using your concentration.
6. As B fills, A empties ... You are Transmuting.
7. When B gets some substance and form, sense outside it along its edge for something around B that is warm ... sense a movement from outside of B into and through it into the emptying Zone A ... now we have motion in both directions, and the transmutation of A is increasing the sense of Emptiness. This is the "Chicken."
8. The Heart Center is present inside the Central Stillness of the Empty Zone A.
9. The Embryo appears, here, then.
10. Zone B becomes global, like a ball rather than an egg shape.

11. Solid Silence can arise (nothing can enter but Love, not even sound).

The energy that creates Zone B comes from leaving "the cave" in Zone A. When we are self-centering, we have a Zone A.

When the Tide centers us, the sense of the body is Zone B suspended and transparent to a Central Stillness in the Sea ... Really.

The chicken allusion is borrowed from *The Secret of the Golden Flower* by Richard Wilhelm with commentary by C. G. Jung ... A chicken sitting on an egg is totally committed, omnipresent to the new chick being formed ... If you have not seen a chicken committed to an egg, you may see this metaphor as weak or silly. The Tide sits and warms us until we hatch. It is a Presence, not a biological force.

The down feathers of a chicken are Warm, Soft, and Embracing ... As is the Presence of the Tide that comes out of the Dynamic Stillness.

The Tide places a mantle around us, and under it we safely unfold. It is The Great Mother of the Womb Creation. It will never leave you. It is Eternal.

The next exercise is helpful because our training in Osteopathic Schools creates good habits that must be abandoned to see into the Midline Therapeutics. Below are common habits that must be reformed.

1st..... Centering down the middle of the patient

This is a subconscious habit of looking down the vertebral column ... is it compressed? Is it straight? When we work with the Fluid, this habit creates a false midline. For some patients, this is overstimulating. For some it is invigorating and they come back for more (become needy). For the Fluid Body itself, it raises the rate (cpm) and opacifies the Zone A (creates tensions). Centering around the edges helps cure this problem.

2nd.....Creating two halves to the body

This subconscious habit believes in left and right sides. So while working, the right hand of the operator palpates one side and the left hand the other, and they are unwittingly juxtaposed around a false midline. The right and left brain are split and the Fluid Body is sheared. This really slows access to the deeper therapeutic forces of Primary Respiration.

3rd.....When we look inside the patient's Zone A for Primary Respiration, we lose the Ocean.

We cut off the Wholeness. We lose the Chicken, the Maternal. We lose the Biodynamics. We create a false wall...This raises the rate and makes us tired.

Outside is the doorway to inside

Inside your head is a cave, a dark cave, where the ego learns to win. In this cave your cleverness cannot be discovered. You can compete and win, unaware of the loneliness you are imprisoned in. You can feel like you are right and others are wrong. Here in the cave, where you sought shelter, is only you. The fear of exposing your nakedness keeps you out of the Sun. The forces against you moving outside are strong. They are alert.

This meditation helps us see the Strength of the forces pulling us inside. We can be patient and compassionate only to the degree that we understand we are all in this boat together, as one broken vessel. Then, it is no shameful thing to be human and to come out and see all the caves on the hillsides. Inside the caves are only small fires, and warm shadows on the wall for company, and dampness as your false Zone B. Find the Health; it is warm.

FINDING CAUSE

Osteopathy was a new science of healing. It did not begin as a subspecialty of Allopathic Medicine. This new science had a unique and effective philosophy that could be applied with skilled senses.

The premise of Osteopathy is that we have the means to heal ourselves. The medicine is and can be manufactured by our own inner resources. Our work with Primary Respiration has proven this premise time and time again.

The principle I wish to address today is "Finding Cause."

In Osteopathy, cause is much deeper than the symptoms ... In Allopathic applications, the symptoms are the cause that one addresses for the cure. However superficial this may appear to any reasonable mind, the fact is that this is the general application of "cure."

All schools of healing in today's Western culture have adopted this mindset that has seeped into all categories of higher education ... including Osteopathy. I can appreciate that superficial symptoms are important to the patient, and I am not proposing that we should not aim to remove the cause of the symptoms ... but what is the Cause?

How deep can one find cause without producing stress on the Whole Patient? Primary Respiration can communicate this to us and is an invaluable tool in helping us Find Cause.

I will focus today on tracking the Cause.

Finding the Cause through history taking is another topic that will be addressed later.

CAUSE, CONTINUED

Our profession is grounded in a unique philosophy and methodology.

We do not believe that the disease is a cause, but a symptom of a deeper disproportion.

We have all heard these words, but most Osteopaths remain unable to see the signs and symptoms presented by the patient as part of a deeper cause that must be addressed. If someone complains of a frozen shoulder, then it is treated as the cause of his or her dysfunction, when in fact we have done nothing to find out why the patient is ill other than be led around by a history that embraces the superficial. The patient says, "I overused my arm doing such and such." The reductionist in us is happy and feels like a real doctor making such superficial connections. This is not Osteopathy.

When I was in Kirksville in 1965, it was impressed upon me over and over again that the symptoms were not the illness. Anyone can make simple conclusions. Anyone can find disease and label it. Still saw into the human organism much more deeply. What was he pointing at, and how do we begin to explore this principle of "finding cause"?

Cause in a reductionistic framework is an isolated force. Effect is what comes from the cause. This is a neat package, except it is not the way nature or life really is. Things do not arise from just the local and present time. The whole life of the patient is the stage upon which insult occurs. Any lesion that is not transmuted remains in us. This lesion is not asleep; it is growing every day in the darkness of our unconscious world.

Lesions are dynamic, they are alive.

They usually grow, and continue to grow, until we meet them

when the Tide brings them into view, at a moment when the whole heals. The power and the timing for the conversion of a lesion comes from the Tide. The power to integrate comes from the reserve we have in the whole. The functional reserve one has is a day-to-day repository. But there could be a lesion draining the reserve as fast as it fills ... this leads to addiction, including addiction to exercise.

Now we will begin to find Cause. The trail is dictated by the Health, which will not let us tread where our logic wants to go. Being a psychologist is of no help here. The Tide will protect the patient from self-criticism while it transmutes the lesion field.

FINDING CAUSE, THE PRACTICAL

Chief complaint ... anything, not just structural.

Find the lesion field ... and the boundary.

Find the force vectors and follow them to the fulcrum.

Pass through the fulcrum, as if it is a doorway.

It will bring you to a new area, a new lesion field.

Go to the area.

Find the boundaries and the force vectors.

Find the fulcrum.

Can you easily pass through the doorway or does the Tide stop your progress?

Continue from place to place until the Tide will not let you through the doorway.

Then treat the patient here, not at the area of the chief complaint.

Recheck in two days.

"It's the not-yet in the now,

the taste of the fruit that does not-yet exist,

hanging the blossom on the bough."

–Laurens van der Post, *Venture to the Interior,*
Harcourt, 1979

FIRST MEDITATION

This morning we are going to "watch" four of the Gifts we are blessed with as a result of being Created.

The Observer

We are given the capacity to observe creation as it occurs.

Generally, the observer is fixed ... unable to be freely shifted by Life as it unfolds. As we saw in Phase Three, the Observer can exhale and become molded (shifted) by the Long-Tide.

There are very great implications to this freedom: a Neutral Heart, Inner Peace, and Love. Consider the reality that you are not your observer. You do not need to observe; it is done for you, like your breathing. Please watch for the automatic shifting of the observer, as a movement of the Tide rather than habit, during this time of meditation. The intrinsic motion of a Free Observer is to be Centered and Stilled by the Breath of Life.

Awareness unfolds like an Embryo.

The Breathing of Thoracic Respiration

Here is something that reveals the nature of our dullness.

We are being breathed, in/out, in/out, with an Intimacy that would shock most people. Right in your own self is a Great Movement of Life ... not a Machine, but a moment-to-moment awakening of your existence. Death/Birth. Repeating a drama that allows Growth and Healing by ending the past and allowing the future only seconds before it too dies.

How far away is the Gift of your being? The Health is not hidden for the elite; it is as near as this breath. We are Living in Intimacy so deep that it may make you a little uneasy.

Just watch the coming and going ... and see the message of a Great Love.

The Sea Around Us

Zone D is the Sea Around Us and Through Us.

Today we are watching this Sea and the Breathing of the Long-Tide. It is an Ocean. In the Shoreline of the Horizon, the Fluid Breathes. It passes through the material world as if it was transparent. The awareness of this is aboriginal; it is normal to feel it. It is spoken of as the Divine Mother in many traditions. The sensation of this Presence is very Intimate and carries with it a sense of Nurture and Shelter. It transforms isolation. One's response is Restful.

SECOND MEDITATION

The Breathing Sea (Zone D), The Breathing Thorax (Zone A), and The Stillness of Zone C

This meditation focuses on the breathing of the Sea (around and through us) and the breathing of Thoracic Respiration, juxtaposed so that we can appreciate their relationship. They originally were one Breath and are trying to return to that Originality. The Stillness in Zone C is related to adoration and devotion to the Divine; it has its own Stillness that is always there. I like to call it crystalline, because it feels like crystal glass. As the three come together, we can see the relationships merge and experience a change in ourselves that leads toward a more concrete awareness of the Health.

Our breathing is usually an effect of our inner state of mind: thoughts, fears, images. Our mental engine is unstable, flitting about, identifying with every movement as "me." We are generally dispersed.

When we bring our attention to the three Landscapes mentioned above, we let the awareness unfold by its own Intelligence. This awareness by itself will follow one landscape then another, automatically shifting, while you just hold your intention to be with the three landscapes, not planning which one to follow. The mind, at a higher level, unites the three into a One, because without our knowing it, this Other-Mind is aware of the Fulcrum around which all three coexist as One.

This Other-Mind will carry you to the Resting Place, a Central Stillness upon which all breath becomes One, and from which it is borne. It is the Health at work in us, guiding the meditation. Sometimes it gets warm.

As we are guided, distractions will enter; do not resist, remain Neutral, let the Tide move the meditation. As The meditation moves along, the rates change in both Primary and Thoracic Respiration, things slow down, the sympathetic tone in us diminishes ... Ease occurs ... the Breathing pauses by itself. We may be breathless for a moment, but something is feeding us, uniting, bringing Stillness into the foreground. Nearer than our breath.

Still, Stilled, Instilled

An Ocean of Center

The Midline that centers us.

Empty the emptiness

Find the Simple

Feel the Liquid Warmth

REFLECTIONS

A wet sponge absorbs water more easily than a dry sponge, and rinses quickly. Slip along your breath into the Interior Castle ... Reflect on these words, paraphrased from St. Teresa of Avila

The Yin and Yang symbol is a circle embracing two fish, one White and one Dark ... some say it is two fishes in the Sea of Life (Zone D). Where is the fulcrum?

We have two self-images; one likes itself and one dislikes itself. This duality is like two mirrors or two facing pages in a book ... when the book folds upon itself, the battle ends and the Book of Life opens. Then the One Image of Self is revealed.

FIRE IN THE BONES

Fire in the Bones Is a Language Developed for Biodynamics.

Fire means potency.

As you know, fire can be of different temperatures, different powers. Fire consumes, as does the potency (i.e., transmutes). The fire is in the waters of life, without being quenched, diminished, used up, or extinguished. It is a Fluid in the Fluid.

The Osteopathic Concept of a "Withering Field" is the foundation upon which we will build our thinking and diagnostics for this practical.

A "Withering Field" is the precursor to disease.

It is an Embryological Segment that is wasting, losing vitality and involuntary motions. This stasis can be appreciated as a dryness, compression, or deformity in a bone or other tissue. We see this frequently in Osteoporosis, chronic postural strains, postsurgical tissue matting … et cetera. The motions vital to healthy tissue, such as venous, arterial, lymphatic, neurotrophic, thoracic, respiratory, and primary respiratory, all arise from protoplasm, and at the Neutral they exchange as One Fluid. As stasis sets up, the Physiology dries out and the Fluid Drive weakens …

The Waters of Life are not irrigating the soil, the fields … in the dry soil the wheat cannot grow, it wilts and eventually withers; if left, it dies. Still was fond of this teaching.

The capacity for neutral, for fluid interchange, and for renewal diminishes … We can feel different levels of decline by trying to feel for the quality of irrigation, the Fluid Drive, the density of the bone, and the response to thoracic respiratory motion.

As your clinical results prove this principle to be true, then we can all begin to think more like Osteopaths, seeking the Potency of Life as a Whole.

As we work with "Fire in the Bones," we will practice using a principle that involves the Long-Tide. This principle will be used again to work with Ignition. Today we are warming up for a greater task.

For the sake of communication I will use steps. Once you are able to be more familiar with these principles, the dimensionality will change and access will become simple.

1st ... Find a "Withering Field."

2nd ... Sense and listen for a Central Stillness in the bone; wait until that Stillness centers you and you are aware of Zone D, without going into it ... This is the key step!

3rd ... Now, find the Long-Tide in the Ocean of Zone D (remember, Zone D is through us as well as outside of us, so do not look very far, just around the edge of the bone).

4th ... Draw the Long-Tide into the bone without disturbing the whole patient.

5th ... Heat will build up and create a warm, ameboid-like shape. Shape your attention and Hands around the shape of the heat, not the bone ... important.

6th ... Continue to relate to the shape of the heat, and again draw the Long-Tide into the shape of the heat ... this creates second-level heat ... the difference between first- and second-level heat is dramatic. Sometimes patients really feel it.

7th ... The second level builds.

8th ... Saturation occurs but may not involve the whole bone ... a variety of end points are possible.

In a sense, we have begun the treatment by directing the Long-Tide, something that raises some interesting thoughts. Fire, at a certain level, can be drawn into a lesion field as a therapeutic force; at other levels "directing" is not possible.

This principle is useful in areas with postsurgical tissue matting (e.g., postmastectomy), remolding of bones after joint replacements, and anytime you find an isolated Withering Field.

PERINATAL OVERVIEW

Prenatal Pelvis

Turning Babies: why do babies turn when we apply Midline principles?

Labor at 36–43 weeks (280 days)

Postnatal

Child

Mother

Family (Zone B, mother, father, child, as One)

Axioms:

"Space opens and function moves in; the path is set by Primary Respiration."

"Do not symmetrize the pelvis."

"Remolding is accomplished by the forces of growth and development (the Fluid Body)."

"Ignition boosts itself with the First Breath; primary and thoracic respiration synchronize."

"Positional shifts in bones after birth are related to Fluid Body activity. There are no biomechanical forces that can accomplish this level of precision and safety."

"Birthing is a CV4. Unfolding occurs naturally through fluid drive. If the fluid drive is low, then the recovery of form and function are delayed."

"The eighty to ninety pounds per square inch of pressure on the child is balanced by the fluid and potency. The tissue forces are inadequate. Think about a newborn with an eighty-pound bag of cement on it, pressing. All that force is enough to rupture the body. Think about this. Next time you're in a hardware store, lift a bag of cement … Feel the force of this amount of pressure."

THE PELVIC BOWL AND THE PERINATAL PERIOD

The process of pregnancy is a Mystery colored by many cultural beliefs. The word "prenatal" means "before being born." In its wholeness, it is a community affair shaped by the Elders and Wisdom keepers. In the Western world, this is lost. There are some exceptions, of course, but most women today face a barren landscape of support that is taxing to their inner world.

This work, using Biodynamic Principles, will prove almost miraculous in its assistance to the work of Nature during pregnancy. In my forty years of practice as Osteopathic GP, nothing has proven Osteopathy more than perinatal treatment.

In this realm, we cannot imagine the Truth that lies often unseen. The sadness is that so many parents, grandparents, elders, and physicians are totally out of touch with the Beauty and Unfoldment of Life during pregnancy. It is most often treated with the same orientation that is used to treat a disease.

This bareness ends up affecting the patient's confidence in their own inner realization of the Mystery of Love. People fear a less-than-perfect progress or outcome. Why?

As practitioners, we must face this void in the culture and be humble enough to be a support system that has Osteopathic thinking at its base.

My plea here is to trust The Ocean Tide and see what happens during treatment and conversation. We cannot change the world, but we can be true to our profession and our patients.

All the issues of abortion, fear of a deformed child, loss of attractiveness, family addictions, support issues, personal capacities, sexuality, sensuality, affection, myths about delivery, financial issues, self- orientation to career, breastfeeding, parenting skills, vaccinations, blood tests, hospitals, and insurances all overshadow the Background of the Movement of Creation. Socrates said, when asked what he did, "I am a midwife ... I help people give birth to their Souls" (paraphrased).

Pregnancy in many cases is about the birth of Being ... for a whole Family.

We all die. When a child comes "in," someone will eventually "leave" ... we must feel more than ourselves at Work if the responsibility of life is to be given over to Life and the Ocean of Palpable Wisdom we call the Tide.

Pregnancy is the period before the birth when it is possible to understand that we are not here to control outcomes, but to respond to the Intention of the Creation ... therein is Peace, Neutrality, Change, Wholeness, and Mystery we can trust.

There is another challenge we must meet in our thinking. Pregnancy is not a biomechanical event. The tissues are not fighting, resisting, and overcoming each other. The changes are all guided by the Fluid Dynamics and the Tide Itself.

Often Osteopaths are trained to think that the changes in form that take place are tissues being forced to yield. Thinking this way is Contra Naturam and leads to less than adequate treatment.

The growth of the child is not biomechanical, we know that ... AND ... neither is the growth of the mother. They are in the Ocean and being shaped by It. The changes in the Child- Mother-Ocean are not segmental, nor are they dictated by somatic activity in the vertebral column, orientated to a notochordal midline.

The activity is Biodynamic in a manner described by Blechschmidt.

The whole changes. The faces, the chests, the abdomens, the pelvises, the viscera, the consciousness, and the persons in the Family circle, even if they appear indifferent.

Treating from a Biomechanical Concept limits the therapeutic potential for the patient. Try to feel the child-and-mother wholeness under the gaze of the Tide. Watch what happens when all three are seen at Once.

For example, the pelvic floor is not stretched out during labor. It happens over months, but not as a stretching. The tissue changes to a moldable jelly. In the gel-like state, a fluid in the fluid opens a new shape. You can see the space open and the form change afterward, just like an embryo. Same Teacher, same School!

You will see the space across the ischia change easily during the last four months. You will see the pelvic floor thin and circumferentially widen. You will see the space between the tents open. You will see the uterus and ovaries travel a great distance, without a war between tissues or visceral combat.

You will see the Long-Tide potentize the uterus and balance the forces on the child during labor; as It opens the doors ... the pain and travail vary with the mother's sense of the Outside Presence that guides the movements ... the mother does not push the uterus ... the tide does. Youhave all seen the force the Tide can generate ... but it also opens the space before its forces easily create change.

Our orientation will be such that you will not see segments or anatomy when the treatment is in process. Why? Because the whole is shifting its wholeness. Tissue follows later.

The Primary Axes of the Pelvic Bowl

Space Opens in a Shape,

Function Moves into the Ease of That Space ... the Birth Canal

THE PELVIC BOWL, PRINCIPLES OF TREATMENT

The principles discussed here originated with Dr. Sutherland. He taught Dr. Ruby Day, my mentor for many years. She began with him around 1935 and continued learning from and teaching with him until his death.

The sitting position we will use today for the treatment of the pelvis was the first thing she did when I went to her for my initial treatment. I had been in pain for fourteen years. No one could help me. I was in practice near her home. I went to seek help for hip pain from a fractured pelvis at age fourteen. She sat me on a table facing her and floated my legs into a position of ease. After two minutes in neutral she said, "Let's see if that helped" ... she was casual in her summation.

I thought to myself, "This is not going to help," but her presence spoke to me unlike any other physician's ever had. Her reputation as a Country Doctor was deeply impressive ... people loved her and she was known to be an excellent Osteopath. Several hours after her treatment, the pain and limp were gone ... forever. I became her student for many years.

She is still here, in this writing and in this teaching.

Before Osteopathy, she was a teacher. Her notes from Will were exact (as were Dr. Wales's). Each visit to her home was an event. She prepared a lesson for each visit, with a concern for detail that I overlooked at first as I hurried to master the "Work," as she called it.

After I took off my self- absorption, she presented a plan for that evening and for "homework." One day, many years later, she said, "I have no more to teach you."

I wanted nothing more than to continue to be in her presence. She was finished. I was heartbroken ... long years of discipline, big challenge, love beyond all of time, all seemed threatened to fade ... they did not. She was a real Teacher, and discharging me was a lesson in detachment for both of us. She died several years later ... What follows is from her effort to preserve the Tradition.

The concept of the pelvis has become divided into Anatomical, Functional, and Biodynamics. Beyond all these academic labels is True Pelvis.

The pelvic bowl treatment, as we approach it, came through Sutherland, probably from Still. The first classes he had, in the thirties, promoted what became know as BMT (balanced membranous tension—there are several varieties) and evolved to where it is today, work without anatomy. I am sure that what we are doing is nothing new for Will Sutherland. The teaching he did was hard because Osteopaths wanted a mechanical approach, and, as Anne Wales and Alan Becker told us many times, "The teaching of the fluids was impossible; many neglected it and could not go further." The outcome of this was the abandonment of the first edition of *Osteopathy in the Cranial Field* for a period of almost forty years.

THE PRINCIPLES OF TREATMENT PRACTICAL

*Begin with the patient sitting, facing you.

*Keep a one-inch space between the patient's knees and the table.

*This allows for automatic shifting to occur more easily.

*Have the patient slump to remove any postural holding.

*Have the patient lean to the right, and slip your right hand under the left pelvis; repeat on the right side ... now, both hands are holding a bowl of "water."

*The ischia are just medial to your hands; you can appreciate them and the space in between. As pregnancy progresses from month to month, this diameter will change ... the tissue will transmute and soften ... these changes are indicators of a normal metabolic shift in the tissue function as it becomes more like a gel.

*Motion testing of the pelvic floor is circumferential, either clockwise or counterclockwise. This simple and effective use of BMT is great for training students. Take a moment and check this, just for review. We will not use the tissue information for treatment.

*Our aim today is to use the Midline as a Therapeutic Agent, so we will sense a bowl of water—no anatomy, no motion testing.

*We then find the Central Stillness, and wait for our consciousness to be shifted.

*Do not "gear up" your effort or attempt to be "present."

*There is an internal Midline and Transverse Axis that one can often see when the mind is awakened by the Tide. If we see these lines, they will be translucent and still, not black and magnetic. If they occur, then find the Central Stillness from which they emerge.

*As you are brought into the treatment there will be no anatomy, only a moldable gel and/or a visceral somatic seam in the whole abdominal-pelvic cavity.

*Once our consciousness shifts, we become aware of the Central Stillness and Zone D.

*A wide, soft, gel-like wave will move slowly around the edges of the area.

*Watch, do not lead.

*If you see anatomy, then you have added too much of yourself.

*Listen to the Whole of Primary Respiration as the local events progress.

*At the end point, everything is homogenized, quiet, still ... no wave is seen.

*Let this maturate, and then check for rebalancing.

Treatment during pregnancy has a lot of power.

If the patient is in labor, she may lean on your shoulders to rest during contractions.

TREATMENT AFTER CENTRAL STILLNESS

The style of treatment that comes after the Central Stillness acts on your awareness and can be "nothing" but a simple movement of Stillness. This activity often begins with an awareness of an encapsulated stillness in the pelvis or abdomen ... like a pool of still water ... Then, instead of a warm gel-like molding process, the Stillness methodically fills all of Zone A , then all of B, then all of C, then all of D ... then ... one senses an incarnate wholeness, and a transparency to the Presence of the Tide, Creation, and Love ... the observer watches this occur ... it seems like so little, so easily ... and it is finished.

The Key Is Letting the Tide Center You

THE CLINICAL HIGHLIGHTS OF TREATING THE PELVIS DURING PREGNANCY

The principles we have explored here are very useful in many situations. Any dysfunction of the pelvic viscera, lymphatic flow, soma, etc., can be approached through the principles we used today.

Prenatal Period

Please remember, we are not visualizing gross anatomy or segmental elements. Any mindset that goes after the lesion directly, to release the somatic tension, will fail to engage the power of the Dynamic Stillness and will not embrace the whole of the patient.

Clinical results are proportionate to the application of principles that do not override the Tide and its Wisdom. This demands discipline on your part not to apply biomechanical principles when using higher laws of healing. This is a hard thing for many people to adjust to.

What you may see, without visualizing, are Seams, the pre-segmental spatial dynamics of the Matrix folding as a whole. During treatment we often see an oval seam between the visceral and somatic functions of the abdomen and pelvis, as a single space.

Treatment from the pelvis changes the dynamics of the viscera (uterus, pelvic floor, prostate, bladder, gut, thoracic abdominal seam, et cetera). During pregnancy, when the patient's adaptive symptoms express urinary frequency, pyrosis, pelvic floor pain, and many other individual problems, this approach really works ... easily.

The treatment feels like a warm gel, molding easily, and in a short time it ends in a Neutral. Be careful not to overtreat. If you do, you will get tired. The treatment takes place around the edges of the visceral sac, but inside the somatic wall ... in a warm, molding, gel-like wave.

Remember the meditation of centering around the edges in oneself, and how that allows a relationship with the Midline and its Potency to express itself? Well, here we are living it.

If you work this way prenatally, you will prevent fetal malposition. Even if you do not deliver babies, you will still find that many people seek out treatment during pregnancy. As you treat some, more will come, because the treatment works.

If the patient does not come until the last weeks of pregnancy, you may think about using the "turning the baby" technique as well as the pelvic bowl approach.

If you read Dr. Still's comments on obstetrics, you will find enough Osteopathic thinking to cure any orthopedic attitudes you might have picked up in your studies. Most health care professionals do not think Osteopathically. We must claim our profession by living it. One of Still's strong suits is his awareness of the Whole as a reality. In his description of balancing the pelvic floor (*Philosophy of Osteopathy*, section on Obstetrics), he engages the "soft parts" above the pubes and the pelvic floor ... He says little ... if this plan is followed during the last trimester ... you will feel the tissue become a gel, really.

When the biodynamic principles noted above are engaged in the manner he describes, the whole perineum is a gel, easily molded toward a new form and physiology (transmutes). Then, as it becomes a syncytium, it homogenizes ... then the movement of thoracic respiration empties itself through the field of the pelvic floor. Something beautiful occurs as a simple, deep Neutral maturates. This helps the bladder adapt; the tissues become a gel and the cervix flattens, softens, and opens. Transmutation is at work.

The reality of tissue becoming gel is, in itself, a truth one can feel. So reread Still and see if his words hold Truth.

Near the seventh month, another phenomenon occurs, demonstrating the principle that Space Opens in The Dynamic Stillness of the Protoplasm, and function moves in, creating form. This is a fact of great importance. It is why we do not recommend trying to make the pelvis symmetrical by manipulating it. During the middle of the third trimester, as you hold the pelvic bowl you will feel a space inscribed in the Fluid Field that marks the space that is opening as a birth canal, into which the child can easily find a pathway (its position for delivery) to the pelvic floor. As the child goes left or right it spirals around the Midline, and when the head arrives in this world it is perfectly centered again, on the midline (sagittal suture centers on pubes). This is quite remarkable to witness, especially if you think birth is a mechanical interface between tissue forces, and that no preparation is anticipated by Mother Nature and her Agencies.

One sees Space open before these events transpire, not during the event itself, by force; the force is only at the final doorway.

All these principles are quite beautiful. They are not created by science ... Nature and the Tide have healed our minds and senses and unveiled something precious to us, and through that witness has come a Tradition. The Science of Osteopathy.

DURING LABOR

The movement of labor receives support and wisdom from many sources. The Long-Tide plays a role in setting the wholeness of the event in motion. It comes from the Sea Around the patient and in some Mysterious way catalyzes the ripening and transport of the mother, child, and father into a new world. If the parents are aware of these things, then the outcome is profoundly spiritual and fulfilling; otherwise, its outcome has a variety of expressions.

The movement in health care today is to think of pregnancy as something to get through, then life, instead of becoming more, is forced to return to its prior pattern. The outcome is that the old pattern demands the organizing of a new form around the old, and the stress levels fly up. This requires some education from us to the patient, but often it is overlooked in the end.

Labor should be supported by someone with insight and the time to commit to the event. Dr. Still believed the Osteopath should stay with the patient throughout. Midwives are excellent. The treatment during labor is to have the patient sit, as in the practical. This position supports fetal momentum, and the mother can rest her arms on one of your shoulders. The treatment will be obvious, as the forces of the Tide are extremely potent and focused.

The treatment is not a routine. It is only necessary if some form of inertia enters the process or the back pain is outstanding. The mother will often find the position restful, and between contractions may rest on the Tide (looks like sleep). Participating in this service is a privilege. It awakens in us Nature's Way and gives us knowledge that is nowhere else to be found but by the Art of Living Osteopathy. The task of "centering around the edges" can help our understanding of the role of the Long-Tide in the movement of birthing, both literally and figuratively. We need the Tide to ripen our consciousness, to place it in a new sensorium.

POSTNATAL TREATMENT

The journey completes itself. Now the forces that created all the growth and change in the mother and child continue to work toward Wholeness. The child enters a new circle. We will discuss this elsewhere.

The mother has a large number of segmental hormonal, mental, and visceral changes. The uterus, for example must change size. It grew all the way up to the size of the diaphragm (ovaries too). Now it returns to the pelvis. The peritoneal "sac" moved along with it. The Fluid Body opened all these changes before the tissue transmuted and changed shape. The shape of the head changed, the upper and lower tents moved dramatically, the pelvic floor turned soft and gel-like, the breasts changed shape. The body fat content shifts, the hormones all move kaleidoscopically, the sense of self shifts, faith increases or decreases, the gut and bladder move around, the liver is busy, the placenta is gone, the immune system readjusts, the heart opens and opens, Zone B becomes communal, et cetera. Who can move all this at once?

There are several highlights from the Biodynamics of *Osteopathy in the Cranial Field* that I would like to note as places that need evaluation. As was noted above, the tents change during pregnancy. If they do not unfold after delivery, the patient can have thyroid dysfunction, headaches, mild hypertension, et cetera. The principle of treatment is the whole, but if that is not forthcoming easily, then one can go to the seam between the tents and find the Long-Tide as we did in Phase Three. The treatment is simple, so do not hang out too long trying to fix tissue. The results are immediate (forty-eight hours or less). Remember that the core of the hormonal system is at the fulcrum of the tents' origin, and they develop as one movement. As the Long-Tide works, it moves everything. That is why, once the treatment starts, no anatomy is visible. The next place to evaluate, if the whole will not respond, is the thoracic-abdominal seam.

THE FIRST BREATH

The first breath of a newborn has always been a moment of marvelous beauty and relief.

In pediatrics texts there are many notable points of evaluation and remedy that one should already know.

This commentary, then, is about Osteopathic vital signs related to this First Breath and how that creates momentum for present and future health issues. Little is written on this subject, but the oral teaching has been passed on for decades.

All the courses I attended mentioned the First Breath. The person who made the most sense to me was Dr. Fulford. He focused on the long-term sequelae in persons who had not completed the First Breath, those who were desynchronized.

Completeness Is Necessary.

The fullness of completion results in a Whole individual aligned consciously and able to function freely. These words coming from Dr. Fulford were few and valued. What did he mean?

My understanding, while talking to him, was based upon knowledge of the mystical path he had followed and what the words *whole, individual, consciously aligned,* and *free-willed* would mean in Sacred Language.

Children are remarkably complete, whole, and free. They unfold from a blueprint of life set at conception. In order for development to unfold continuously, one must have a well-established fulcrum between Primary Respiration, Thoracic Respiration, and Ignition.

At the time of First Breath, the demands of life are increased severely ... the Ignition creates more fire, the Long-Tide is orchestrated, the Dynamic Stillness pours in through the Midline, and as the air rushes into the lungs, One Breath is set in time as Eternity comes ashore.

This would be my understanding of the Wholeness that Dr. Fulford mentioned to me in 1979.

To be an Individual, in Dr. Fulford's terminology, means to follow the destiny of unfoldment, not worldly images. The journey for Dr. Fulford was to listen to the Love behind Creation and follow Its voice. The result of this hard work would be to become what God made one for, not what one's genetics and ego might overlay.

The First Breath establishes Memory and the vital Oneness that carries one's Name. If the First Breath is weak, our struggle to know ourselves may be extended and spiritual maturity delayed (prolonging the sense of isolation).

To be Consciously Aligned means, in the context of his work, to be aware of Divine Will and to have an instinctual need to be in the presence of Love and Perfection.

Free will, as Dr. Fulford put it, is when One has no slavery to habits or beliefs. One is free to be shifted by the movement of the Creator's Hand. One is free to lighten the load of world suffering. One is detached, impartial to everything, and responsive to the unfoldment of God's love. This is not "willy-nilly," going with the flow ... it is love meeting Love with no preconceived outcome.

It is fearless in the face of one's lesions.

In the Biodynamic View, the First Breath Is Relative.

The First True Breath is at or before conception. Obviously, thoracic respiration (0_2 metabolic exchange) begins much earlier than birth.

The Presence of Primary Respiration guiding conception is a Biodynamic Principle that emerges from both Osteopathy and Embryology.

The Birthing Breath is the first earthly breath and, ideally, thoracic, primary, and the Ignition move together as One. The diagnostics around this are covered in Pediatrics Phase Two.

Think about the capacity of Zone B to do its work, to accomplish unfoldment of the blueprint of Life if the First Breath is desynchronized and weakened.

The first hint of this, if you are not trained to see it through fluid body dynamics, is slowness in the remolding of the head after birth. This should be a red flag that there is a problem in the Core.

At conception the Divine Image is Breathed into protoplasm (clay). The perfect image is made; we call it the Health. This is a lifelong reference point for normal that is indispensable for healing and unfoldment. Without this, life does not move forward, it terminates. Protoplasm is the first moldable substance that can hold an image, and the image is unerring in its timing and geometry. The inscription is Immortal.

This could be called The Absolute First Breath.

Reflection on this surpasses the written history of human life.

Each of us must think about this truth in the light of the clinical and personal outcomes we experience day to day in our work.

BIRTH

Fire ... Ignition ... O_2 *... Dynamic Stillness ... All Breathe*

The Child ... One Breath ... Incarnation Unfolds.

THE NEWBORN

Biodynamics offers several courses focused on the treatment of newborns. The time frame in Phase Four limits our work to Midline Therapeutics only.

A newborn for our purposes is a child up to age one.

Midline orientation is absolute in the development of healthy milestones. This includes several aspects of Perception ... general awareness, horizontal fixation of the ocular-vestibular-cephalic reflex, immune centering and discernment, attention flexibility, and bonding (Zone B).

We are only as functional as our Midline relationship.

For a child, Zone B is a collective "body." It includes both parents and other Family members ... keep this in your awareness as you are treating!

Children Do Not Feel a Zone A Unless Traumatized.

Several Kinds of Treatment Will Be Demonstrated:

Long-Axis release of fluid body

An easy and very effective release of the crown-to-rump compression from labor, using brief direct and prolonged indirect actions in relation to the Fluid Body.

False and True Midline relationship

A simple, effective way to reestablish the relationship between Soma and true Midline.

Inversion

Allows the Fluid Body to Unwind in the Sea; the child will translate in space.

Inversion was accidentally discovered by Stuart Korth and me, independently of each other. It has been used thousands of times by both of us, and by many other clinicians.

It involves turning the infant upside down while holding the pelvis. This, of course, was the child's position for much of the time in utero. It seems natural to the child, but sometimes onlookers may wonder what we are doing. Explain it to them. The child will gyrate in space with great force that may surprise you, so hang on more than you think is necessary, keeping the Child close to you.

The child will show no signs of stress until near the Stillpoint, when it may cry easily for a moment as the birth memory is transmuted.

Then, as the child comes to Neutral, it will make a soft cooing sound, a little "Om." It is quite remarkable.

At the Stillpoint, the air is charged with a sense of peace, and the child is suspended contentedly.

The power present in the gyrations is a real lesson in the tidal forces that hold life. I have never repeated this a second time.

Motion testing the reciprocal tension potency (RTP)

Does it move easily in both directions? This tells us if the Fluid Body has a good range of compensatory function ... this of course determines how well one meets stress of any kind ... It is also an index of the capacity for Neutral (change).

The First Breath

Was it One movement? See commentary on the next page. Is the Ignition adequate?

Children lesion as a Whole. As we mature as Osteopaths, this reality will replace many of our anatomical concepts.

There are other factors to consider that are helpful, but as a first treatment this is enough.

Birthing

Birth is a CV4; the compressive forces are 80-100 psi. After birth, the Fluid Body reshapes and repositions everything in an EV4-like process.

The Fluid Body needs good Ignition to supply the force (fluid drive) for reshaping.

THE MIDLINE

The Midline is a story that will change a great deal as you exchange with it.

The idea of a Midline separate from the notochordal midline or the gravitational midline did not appear in Embryology or Osteopathy until its introduction in the Biodynamic model in 1982.

Our linear concepts of what a Midline is will change in magnitude as we gain experience by working with it. Then we will see something quite Whole, and beyond the laws of simple geometry. The Midline of Wholeness is unerring and perfect in its format; it is a place, not a line.

We must also remember that we see the Midline in a compromised state of expression, because the patient, we ourselves, and our basic education veil the Great Wholeness that is indwelling in the Divine Geometry of Life, Creation, Renewal, and Healing. To see the Midline in a perfect system is to understand the Wholeness of Creation and Life as a singular event.

What we shall see are the lesions that limit midline expression, and we must learn how to treat them. Remember, we are working with broken systems. This does not mean that the Midline can lesion. What we do have is false midlines (compensations), and these can be mistaken for The Midline. Therefore, one foundational task is to discern the difference between the true and false midlines. One aspect of knowing the difference is the effect of what we see upon our own consciousness ... this has great meaning.

As we are, we are restricting the Movement of Creation. This is nothing to be upset or alarmed about, but it is the reason that we and the patient experience things the way we do. Many people have asked me and have promoted the idea that the Perfect Midline is in the perfect location, inside of us (i.e., Zone A). It is not. If we are with the Health, then we shall find its magnitude.

The True Midline does not express anatomy separate from Wisdom; therefore, one should be careful about premature knowledge that is misleading. When we are conscious enough, the Perfect will reveal Itself. Our aim here is to understand the lesioning process and disorientation of anatomy in ourselves and the patient as having moved away from the Healthy True Midline.

We have already seen some expressions of Midline function when we studied the Axial Fluctuations and the "fluid in the fluid" in Phase Two. We saw that the potency (reciprocal tension potency, fluid in the fluid, fire) seems to arise from the center and move toward the periphery as it creates the form of Zone B. The fire that builds us has an indwelling Wisdom that brings not just power but also form, function, and perfection into each breath. When it is free to express itself, it transmutes our lesions (Zone A) and creates a Zone B. We saw this in our meditation and in treatment.

THE FUNCTIONS OF THE MIDLINE

The most important principle in Phase Four is that The Midline "centers" us.

This requires that we be Neutral and let the Midline center us ... how long does this take ... seconds ... how do we know ... we see our mind shift its awareness to where the TIDE takes it ... the Sea of Stillness. This unveiling is Given, not taken, by our own power.

We can believe that we are more conscious than others. The symptoms of this illusion are loneliness, false humility, impatience with others, belief that our belief is correct for everyone ... therefore, we will miss the diversity of Wholeness and the Charity of Understanding. In other words, we are not freed by being "centered," but imprisoned by willpower. What is only acquired by the Generosity of Creation cannot be owned. What we take by force does not bring Peace, only more subtle suffering. Being Centered by the Tide removes a great burden from one's shoulders ... we realize that we are not the Center of knowledge and being ... we are an expression of Life ... this includes being powerless to control the Indwelling forces of Healing beyond the level of symptomatic relief. We begin, as always, with the Healthy Functions ... Here, because we are moving beyond rates, we make an effort to sense (listen for) the Dynamic Stillness at the center, instead of anatomy. We listen with our hands for a Stillness, and no other phenomena (Fluid body, et cetera). When we hear it, by listening in different ways until it is unveiled, our awareness is moved by the Mechanism to the Sea Around Us ... we become centered by the Tide (i.e., synchronized). The task here is not to go out to Zone D but to be taken into a shift in awareness that takes us into An Ocean of Stillness ... this is the key to exploring the Midline Functions ... We do this synchronization for the same reason as in other Phases, that is, to not disturb or lesion the patient with our attention to lesions and Allopathic principles.

When we enter The Sea Around Us, it is Silent and Full. We are no longer aware of the Long-Tide or rates. We are in the Dynamic Stillness. Once we have synchronized, several functions of the midline can be appreciated.

Midline
Dynamic Stillness
Ignition, light, warmth
Potency, Dynamic Stillness
Potency, reciprocal tension potency moving around the core as a Zone B
Reciprocal tension potency in lesion, Zone B is restrained as a compressed field of reciprocal tension potency
Light fire, ignition, Spark of Life
Spatial Alignment of Form and Function (growth, healing, renewal, and automatic shifting)
Segmental Organization (secondary midline)
Synchronization of the parts to the Whole (during treatment this happens during pauses)
Reflects the Oneness of Nature, Life, and the Divine
Generation of life forces and axial fluctuations
Acts as a "Single Fulcrum" suspended in the Sea around Us
Core-Link
Doorway for Therapeutic Power
Center of the Health
Transformer ... converts rates
Wisdom is an Immune Function
Residual compensatory relation with lesions
Wholeness

Functions without Autonomic Polarity (sympathetic/parasympathetic), trophic

Center for all Zones and the Link beyond to the Stars

Cannot lesion

Not the line of gravity, nor is it the midline of Polarity Therapy

During the practical, we will see only some of the above. Please note there is no Zone A.

THE MIDLINE, PRACTICAL ONE

Make observations at different sites (cranium, thorax, feet, coccyx). If nothing comes easily, move on to another place. Do not force your attention. Let the Central Stillness transmute your awareness and open the landscape.

Make sure the patient is in Neutral on the Long-Tide or Dynamic Stillness. If not, either wait or rebalance the patient.

Make notations of what aspects you see easily and which are vague. Remember, there will be no anatomy used for this Phase.

Things of interest:

The Central Stillness: once you sense it, it transforms your mind to The Ocean around and through the patient.

Light: soft, liquid light that is central.

Both of the above are aspects of the Health.

Blackness around the core Health: this is restricted reciprocal tension potency, from sympathetic overtones.

Life Force: the movement of Something through everything, as if everything was transparent life force: soft potency.

The Sea Around Us: a full Zone D and more.

Space without anatomy, segments, or rates, just a stillness, and a moldable substance.

Finally, review the Long-Tide and the Midline... be aware of the Long-Tide in Zone D and the coccyx as a doorway. As the Long-Tide comes toward the doorway and you are with the Central Stillness, what transpires?

... If one focuses on anatomy, it can lesion the area around the midline (reciprocal tension potency) even more ... The patient may feel confined, startled, have palpitations, have a desire to run away, or other kinds of instinctual responses.

Once you are seeing something important, do not let your mind become absorbed in it. If this happens, do not back off … simply go to the Central Stillness, and wait for the anatomy to disappear.

If the patient continues to react, go to the cisterna chyli and find the Long-Tide; wait and follow the Direction of Ease.

MIDLINE FUNCTIONS

The Midline Centers Us

When we touch the Midline, it transmutes our awareness, and we become aware of Zone D. This often occurs so quickly that you can miss it, because of your expectations of time. Try to see the immediacy of Change. Study the shift in the space and motion as it is changed by the Potency of the Midline. The Midline is a Central Stillness; as you sense it, there is a change in consciousness.

Once we have been synchronized by the Central Stillness, several functions of the midline can be appreciated.

Midline

Dynamic Stillness

Ignition, light, warmth

Potency, Dynamic Stillness

Reciprocal tension potency moving around the core of the Midline as Zone B

Reciprocal tension potency in lesion, Zone B is compressed; the field of reciprocal tension potency is clinging to the center, giving the appearance of a black line (false midline)

Light, fire, ignition, Spark of life

Spatial Alignment of Form and Function (growth, healing, renewal, and automatic shifting)

Segmental Organization (secondary midline)

Synchronization of the parts to the Whole (during treatment, this happens during pauses)

The Oneness of Nature, life, and the Divine

Generation of life Forces and Axial Fluctuations

Acts as a Single Fulcrum, suspended and Shifting in the Sea around Us

Core-Link

Doorway for therapeutic power

Center of the Health

Transformer ... converts rates

Centers the Immune Function

Residual compensatory relation with lesions

Functions without Autonomic Polarity (sympathetic/parasympathetic), trophic

Center for all Zones

Cannot lesion

It is not a Line of gravity, nor is it the Midline of the Polarity, as described by Stone, D.O.

Please note there is no Zone A.

During the practical we will see only some of the above. Give yourself a year to complete the list.

THE MIDLINE, PRACTICAL TWO

This practical attempts to reinforce the understanding that the Midline has a direct relationship to soma, and that when soma lesions that relationship remains intact...

It seems difficult for Osteopaths to adjust to the reality that somatic position is not a by-product of biomechanical forces. It is even more difficult to imagine that positional corrections can be accomplished by the Fluid Body. Soma also has a positional response to the Dynamic Stillness of the Midline. How is this possible?

Think about babies turning in the uterus after being really stuck in fetal malposition. How is it that babies turn without the usual mechanical forces, applied with straps, and how do they turn with the Principles Applied?

We are approaching the question: can an Osteopathic lesion shift position without fluid forces or direct or indirect action?

The practical is easy. The principles are easy, but what is the means by which we can explain these activities? ...

Begin with the Sacrum.

The Sacrum has many kinds of normal motion. Do multilevel diagnosis first, then we can see how much change does or does not occur, using the suggested principles.

Is there a positional restriction ... Remember, there are translational lesions.

Is there a response to Thoracic Respiration? ... Does it move the sacrum or pass through it?

Is there a response to Primary Respiration? ... toward lamina terminalis, during the Inhalation Phase of Primary Respiration.

Does the tide suffuse the bone and transmute it (i.e., intraosseous breathing)?

Are all the segments moving? Are any segments lesioned (positionally or as "Withering Fields")?

The treatment is to let go of all information, sense the Central Stillness, and wait for your mind to shift (it may take only a millisecond, so watch carefully).

Is there a shift in position as a result of Midline Therapeutics?

Our next stop is at C7.

To give us a fuller understanding of principles, the approach here is a little different than with the Sacrum.

Sit at the side of the patient.

Find the spinous process and the two transverse processes of C7. The upper hand is posterior, and the lower hand is bridging the neck and perching on the transverse processes (in a large neck just project the sensing).

Without using anatomy, find the Central Stillness, and wait as before. What transpires? Does soma move?

Rebalance the Patient Before Going to the Next Area.

THE ATLAS

The history of this bone is interesting and should be reviewed. Its growth, ossification, muscular attachments, and neurophysiology are all important.

During extension injuries, the Occiput wedges forward into the convexity of the two kidney bean–shaped facets of the upper surface, known as the Atlas. As it passes its physiological barrier, the intraosseous matrix of the Atlas bends. The intraosseous bending is such that the anterior tubercle moves forward as the transverse processes move posteriorly and medially.

The small muscles of the cranial base go "haywire." The ocular-cephalic-vestibular mechanism is overloaded and the muscles contract.

The results are severe and easily become chronic. The Atlas locks around the condyles as the muscles tense and cast the lesion into inertia. As time passes, the bones mold into deformity. This is not a Biomechanical lesion. The tissue fluid and potency are locked up in a lesion field that extends from the eyes to T4.

The ease of treatment with Midline Dynamics is cause for reflection. A "bad lesion" does not mean you try harder.

The Atlas is a place where a great deal of geometry intersects

*A line from the premaxilla through the anterior tubercle and the posterior arch (if the bone is perfect)

* A transverse line across the transverse processes (if they are perfect)

*A vertical line through the odontoid (if the segment is perfectly on the notochordal midline). All this is a picture of Health ... so how do we use the Midline Therapeutics to approach the Atlas?

First, every lesion is imperfect; the lesion never fits the descriptors exactly. As Rollin once said to me, as I tried to see every detail of a lesion, "If you keep learning and seeing more, you will see that the true lesion field could only be appreciated if you had a computer, and ten years to find all the strains." He was absolutely correct!

We can become overloaded and overwhelmed by knowledge. We need the Wisdom of the Tide to sort this out, and as it does you will learn a lot about the formation of lesions as well as the Health, which brings it back toward Midline.

First find the morphology of the lesion field ... then let the anatomy go.

Go to a Central Stillness ... watch your mind shift.

What transpires?

Can you see the bone unbend?

After the end point, listen to the brainstem ... how is everything?

Rebalance, if needed.

THE UNIVERSALITY OF THE MIDLINE

The Midline is Everywhere, expressing the Architect that Moves the "Whole." This is a Midline for the Health.

We have submicroscopic and macroscopic Midlines.

There are segmental midlines, bodily midlines, individual midlines, et cetera. There are Collective midlines (mother, father, and child, for example).

There are Midlines for Humanity (C. Jung, M.D.)

There are Midlines for Conscience (van der Post, *The Face Beside the Fire*)

The Midline and Zone B form shelter.

There is a nongenetic Family Midline and a Family Midline.

There are Tribal Midlines.

Every Rate has a Midline.

There are False Midlines.

All Midlines Link Together

THE BIRD. THE THIRD VENTRICLE. THE INSTINCT AND THE IMAGINATION

The "Bird" is an image set forth by W. G. in his famous teaching "The Tour of the Minnow" to describe the dimensionality of the Third and Fourth ventricles.

The Bird, as an image related to the CV3, was introduced to the profession in 1992 as a special form of Instinctual activity related to the immune system's "coming to Neutral." Shortly thereafter, the precautions were not heeded by some, who insisted on forceful CV3.

The Biodynamic teaching was original work connected to research done in practice by Dr. Blackman and me on CV3 and the Anterior Dural Girdle. The precautions we prescribed have not been universally heeded, so let us begin with a warning.

"A little learning is a dangerous thing; Drink deep, or taste not the Pierian spring" (front page, 1st edition, Osteopathy in the Cranial Field).

Do not use direct action on the third ventricle.

Do not use direct action on the tissue of the anterior dural girdle.

Do not use direct action on the cerebrospinal fluid in the third ventricle.

Do not use direction on the reciprocal tension potency in the third ventricle.

Why not? The risk is very high! ... other techniques are more effective ... and any neurophysiologist will tell you we do not have a map of the Brain. We have almost no understanding of the Mind. The need to manipulate the Natural World is a human shortcoming ... we are responsible for our actions.

Direct action causes subliminal emotional imbalances that are not felt by the patient during the treatment but slowly emerge over months or years and are irreversible emotional liabilities unless treated Biodynamically by someone with many years of experience.

Interviewers who have asked me about this continue to write and teach the opposite, even though it has been stated to them multiple times. Even articles that were corrected by me, at the author's request, were then changed back to a mechanical view in the final draft. I have never taught anyone to manipulate the third ventricle, period.

The task of allowing Neutral in the third ventricle is the goal of anyone who understands Sutherland's work. The CV3 is not focused on the respiratory control centers as the CV4 is, but rather it focuses on the Core of the neuroendocrine immune system, the centers for instinct and deep emotional awareness (subconscious). There is so much here one must admit some humility. So first one must ask, What is this treatment for? Why am I doing this?

Applying techniques to the third ventricle based on symptoms and engaging tissue will not, in the long run, benefit the patient. The Instinct is millions of years old ... to direct or restrain it is a serious misunderstanding of neurophysiology, psychology, states of consciousness, and the power of the Tide.

Anatomy disappears once you go beyond the rate of two to three cycles per minute. The Instinctual operates at the Long-Tide and beyond. Therefore, seeing anatomy when one treats means that one is not synchronized with the level of activity that is necessary for the Neutral to be easily established within the function one is looking at.

We are trying to allow the third ventricle to come to REST. This is the most important function of the immune system and the subconscious. The educated mind is in no way superior to the mind of the "old brain." It is not intelligent to force Nature to respond. She will compensate, and that could mean serious mental fragility for the patient.

Will Sutherland almost died learning CV4. He did not experiment on patients. He was interested in thoracic respiration coming from the deepest possible Neutral, because he saw that state as profoundly healing. He was exploring. He chose V4 for its relationship to thoracic respiration.

He made errors. He learned not to use force. The legacy is ours if we wish. The outcome of his errors was "get as far away from physical touch as possible." (W.G.S.)

He did not force treatments (see April 12, 1948, in Contributions of Thought). The mental shift to a full understanding of this requires humility, submission to a greater Mind, and a Teacher that watches over you, so you do not fail to see your attitudes clearly.

We should be careful that we don't sacrifice the whole to fix the part.

This work is exceptional, but we must learn to communicate with Nature, not control her as Allopathic Medicine does.

As Dr. Sutherland begins "The Tour of the Minnow," he asks us to use our Imagination. What does this word mean to you?

In today's technical world, the word imagination has negative connotations. It is looked down upon by intellectuals and often used to intimate that a person in touch with Imagination is psychologically unstable.

Sutherland was a journalist, a word expert. He chose his words with precision.

Imagination is "the genius of the creative faculty of the mind at its highest aspect."

This does not mean thinking and doing, it means something more essential. The Imagination of children worries some psychologists. The Imagination of elders is written off. We are trained not to trust it in ourselves.

If one empties oneself of what one knows and follows the Imagination, it opens doors to a Reality that supersedes the knowing of popular science, and leads to a knowing that is Neutral, Still, and unquestionable, even if the conditional mind says it's not true.

Our great teachers were not afraid to challenge themselves. Imagination is reached only by denying oneself the expertise of modern thinking and stepping into allusions (not illusions) that soon become principles of living and treatment. Sutherland did so in the "Tour." As we see into the story, the truth proves itself in practice.

Beyond Imagination is the direct sense of the Divine. Memory living in Eternity. All this is connected with the Health inside of us. At each level, new mental activities are accessed.

Sutherland's request to use Imagination must be explored in a serious manner.

The demand that everything must meet the methods of popular scientific research is a narrow belief system, not an objective reality.

The Art of Osteopathy precedes the Science of Osteopathy.

The Bird and the third ventricle are the Wisdom of millions of years of Living. They have a data bank, a growing Memory of Life that sees beyond anything you can be trained to become, but it does not exceed who you Are, in your Health.

IGNITION

Fire is and always has been a precious element of Life. The Engine of Life and its Spark were realities for Dr. Still. Dr. Sutherland continued Still's appreciation for Fire.

Fire is necessary.

Fire is vitality.

Fire keeps our metabolic processes alive, which creates another fire that dies in the caloric burn.

Fire is the Spirit of Primary Respiration, creating the Wholeness of Life.

Fire catalyzes the Breathing of rates and creates the Shape of respiration.

Fire is the Light of Consciousness and Wisdom in traditional stories.

Fire is the Passion of Devotion, of trusting the Tide.

Fire burns, Transmutes lesions, but does not diminish its reserve. Fuel is warmth, the Generosity of a Charitable Heart.

Fire is light that Sees.

Fire is the keeper of the Lamp that lights our way.

Fire consumes the dross, leaving the gold (Health).

Fire creates Fluid Drive.

Fire Generates the Longitudinal Fluctuation, spreads laterally as the Lateral Fluctuation.

Fire is Everywhere at once, but centers itself on the Midline.

IDENTIFIABLE TERMINOLOGY

Breath of Life

The animating essence of Life, Divine Love

Life

"The slow vivifying force moving forth from Deity," "The substance that fills all the spaces of the universe." –A. T. Still

Spark of Life

Fire from the Divine, Omnipotent Fire

Ignition

Transmutation, liquid light, everywhere at once, charges the battery; see "The Tour of the Minnow"

Engine of Life

The singularity of Wholeness, moving as One. The Mechanism. A language introduced by Still

Motion

Movement in time or Eternity

Dynamo

Direct and alternating currents, translates fire into motion, creates a pattern of coiling and uncoiling in reciprocal tension potency (see *Osteopathy in the Cranial Field,* first edition)

Transmutation

$E = MC^2$, $EM = C^2$, EM as One; the complete change in essence ... power and form are one

Metabolic Motion

The effects of transmutation depend upon the Fire. As we saw in Phase One, transmutation creates internal disengagement, internal augmentation, synchronization, neutral, and reorientation of the parts to the whole (Midline). This indwelling capacity for self-correction is the Basis of Osteopathy as Still described it.

Form

Fire has the Intelligence of design. It creates form, even the notochord.

"The Tour of the Minnow"

At the center of the third ventricle is the Fulcrum.

Rates

Compensatory inhalations and exhalations, formed from the fire

Battery of Life

Cerebrospinal fluid as a battery, charged through the fulcrum in the third ventricle by Fire

Tropism

The functional reserve to meet and transform the metabolic effects of stress and create homeostatic neutral. A better word may be *trophicity,* which does not exist. The "Withering Fields" are nourished by trophicity, which is a capacity for neutral at the individual cellular level.

Milestones

There is ignition daily at sunrise, at conception (or before), at the first Breath, at Menopause, at Death, and during Miracles ... each time there is Love in the Fire.

The above language is from Still to Sutherland; exact definitions are not recoverable.

RELATIONSHIPS

DIVINE SPARK -- the spiritualization of matter

SPARK, FIRE -- luminosity, power, life force

SPARK, MIDLINE -- generator, transformer, rates, life force

FIRE, AIR -- metabolism, two breaths meet

FIRE, FIRE -- transmutation

FIRE, WATER -- Fluid Body... protoplasm

FIRE, EARTH -- form, death, birth, humus (humility)

FIRE, SOUL -- awareness, consciousness, Psyche, Eros, Agape, Wisdom, Vision

WHOLENESS -- Eternity incarnates everywhere

In Phase Three we studied the "Bird." The millions of years ... the wisdom of Nature inside of us, Watching. This vigilant instinct is at the core of the immune system. As we saw, it is wiser than we are, and it does not trust human nature as it is. The Bird watched our attitude and was not going to rest until we demonstrated that we could hold our attention on the Stillness of the fulcrum.

When the Bird did rest, it rested upon the Dynamic Stillness of the Sea Around Us. This, of course, is the Dynamic Stillness we are exploring in Phase Four. The Bird is an old Symbol, perhaps from the sages who saw its form in themselves. It has great meaning for many traditions. This is discussed elsewhere.

The reciprocal tension potency in the third ventricle will be our primary interest in Phase Four.

With that orientation, we are not relating to tissue in any manner. This would be dangerous. As we discovered in Phase Three, the Bird is not going to Neutral until we demonstrate that we can be present to the Fulcrum and not place demands on the System.

Our diagnostic question in Phase Four is about whether or not the reciprocal tension potency is "fired up" ... whether it is in a raw state of inertia or whether it is transmuting (moving from the center to the periphery).

Is the ignition creating fluid drive and vivifying the cerebrospinal fluid? Is the third ventricle metabolically able to create neurotrophic flow or not?

Is the reciprocal tension potency moving from the center to the periphery, creating and sustaining Zone B? Is an adequate febrile response possible to pathogens?

Sometimes the third ventricle is dark, there is no sign of light. It feels condensed like a black hole ... this is inertia ... a Lesion Field.

Sometimes the reciprocal tension potency has aberrant motion that turns inward on itself without moving from the center to the periphery. All of these are non-anatomical findings. Tissue and fluid are both showing signs of failure (eczema, fibromyalgia, asthma, autoimmune symptoms) as a result of poor Ignition.

Please understand that low ignition is reflected through the loss of transmutation in all structural and functional involuntary movements.

The Ignition is at the core of the neuroendocrine-immune system. It includes perceptual orientation because the Ignition is a Midline function. As it provides Fire, it also provides spatial orientation for the attention to relate to the horizon.

Osteopathically, when the Ignition is low, we find low fluid drive, loss of axial fluctuations, condensation of intraosseous motion, condensation of the reciprocal tension potency, loss of central nervous system coiling and uncoiling in the brain and brainstem, and increase in the overall rate, until the system eventually fails. Then it recedes to the Ocean, and the patient's psyche is adrift from this world (dissociation). One can sense that the fulcrum for the attention is not in the brain, but outside in the Sea or the Stars.

Neutral is not forthcoming until the Ignition is reestablished ... this can take more time if the origin of the problem is iatrogenic.

Conditions that have been cured in my practice by repeated use of this:

Asthma
Eczema
Postpartum hypothyroidism
Loss of sweating response
Rheumatoid syndromes
Febrile dysfunctions
Systemic lupus
Chronic fatigue
Autisms
Post-immunization paralysis
Failure to thrive
Limb growth delay
Severe neurological dysfunction from placenta hemorrhage
Metrorrhagia
Drug toxicity
Infertility
Grief, true and sustained
Sphenobasilar symphysis compressions are ignition failures, until proven otherwise

IGNITION PRACTICAL

Evaluation of the Ignition Status at the Third Ventricle

We are not looking at anatomy, but rather the state of the reciprocal tension potency and the ease of its activity. Normal function would demonstrate movement from the center to the periphery, fulfilling Zone B. This would mean that the Fire of Ignition is present and free to transmute. The reciprocal tension potency generates motion, vitality, centering, heat, and light (soft, warm). The awareness of these activities comes from letting yourself be aware of a Central Stillness, then it will center you in the "Sea of Stillness." The Central Stillness is not located by using anatomical landmarks.

Often, but not always, there is a sense of an egg-shaped stillness inside the Stillness of the Whole Head. This is the fulcrum of the third ventricle, through which all the embryological and ignition forces emerge. Do not stare.

Next, locate the Long-Tide. Is it penetrating the Stillness of the third ventricle and creating activity.

If the Long-Tide and the reciprocal tension potency are not mingling, then we will most gently embrace the periventricular Long-Tide (part of Zone D) and ...

Bring us into the third ventricle through an opening of ease, like we did with "Fire in the Bones." There should be NO BARRIER.

In severe cases, one may have to use a longer lever, and wait longer.

First-stage heat will now appear.

Wait. As the first heat comes, it has a shape; as you see the shape, let your hands mold sweetly to the form of the heat.

When the shape stops growing, bring the Long-Tide in again ...

The Second-stage heat should begin.

When the Long-Tide saturates the third ventricle to the capacity of the moment, or the Tide tells you, you are done.

What is the final shape that the heat expresses?

Rebalance or Not?

Note: There are a variety of Luminosities that accompany the second-level heat. Sometimes we see a soft warm glow, and other times we see firelight in one, or several, of the following places: the third ventricle, the area of the cisterna chyli, the heart, the pelvic fulcrum, or the Whole of Zone B.

THE WIRE

The Wire is a term used by Dr. Becker in the article "Be Still and Know." The exact meaning he intended is lost in time, but as we worked with the Long-Tide in Phase Three and the Midline in Phase Four, certain activities appeared to be "Wire-like."

This raised the question, "Is this what Dr. Becker was alluding to?"

Also, conversations with his good friend Jacques Duval, D.O., in Paris were helpful, as Jacques felt that Dr. Becker was pointing in the direction that we are discussing.

You will certainly see for yourself.

The Longitudinal Fluctuation associated with the Fluid Body at two to three cycles per minute is following a pathway on the long axis of the Fluid Body. It is oriented to and by something Will Sutherland mentioned in the "The Tour of the Minnow." He imagines a "quiver" coming up the Center.

Current day Embryology is searching for a "centroid" for the movement "Wholeness in the Embryo."

Dr. Becker asked me the question, "How many ways can you spin a ball?" ... "One," he said. "Around its center point."

The Fine-Tuning Techniques and the Power Points Method of Dr. Sutherland both use the Midline for the therapeutic process.

When coming from the horizon to express a treatment, the Long-Tide moves along a distinct line (wire). It, like the Longitudinal Fluctuation inside the Fluid Body, is a long axial movement in the Sea around Us. One is the Long Axis in Zone B, and another is in Zone D.

During Phase Three we let our attention exhale, let it leave our mind. By itself, it headed to the Horizon ... then there was a long pause followed by Something coming over the horizon like a waterfall. Then it changed form, into a linear vector traveling on an axis (wire). It came toward the patient and the operator. They both received treatment.

As we study the Midline and see its dimensionality, we sense "A Wire for Creation."

When we hear the sweet voice of the Presence of the Breath of Life ... we are in touch with the Master. One could say we are on the "Wire," alluding to Communion.

The "Sweet Wire" ... C. Sullivan, D.O.

The "World Axis" ... C. Jung, M.D.

The Bridge Between Worlds, a Meeting Place for Communication with Children

The Earth Has Many Midlines (Gravity, Rotational, Solar, Polar, and Galactic)

The "Axis of Continuum" from Birth to Death

The Central Nervous System Bows Upon It as It Drinks from the Waters of Life (Paraphrased, W.G.S.)

Let's wait for more ...

THE IMMUNE SYSTEM, THE THIRD VENTRICLE, AND THE NEURAL TUBE

This is the beginning of our study of the Immune System, and it will continue throughout all the remaining Phases.

Dr. Still certainly noted the activities of the Immune System ... his ideas included the following:

The Engine of Life

The Spark

Ignition

Fire

Nerve Force

Nerve Flow

The Laws Not Framed by Human Hands

Fever as an Electric Phenomenon

The cerebrospinal fluid (as a Primary Command Post)

The Indwelling Wisdom of The Health

The Eternal as the True Self

Statements like "There Are Finer Nerves Dwelling in the Lymphatics Than in Your Eye" (Paraphrased)

William Sutherland continued to use the language of Dr. Still, which many took as metaphorical daydreams, having never applied and tested the validity in clinical practice of what Still was concretely pointing at.

Still's ideas emerged from observations of Natural Laws at work in his patients and the world around him. Sutherland followed Still's insights and slowly built a framework for Primary Respiration.

Sutherland explored involuntary motions in the central nervous system (CNS) and wrote beautifully in his treatise "The Tour of the Minnow" and other commentaries. Because of these two men, our ability to treat immune problems has developed into a meaningful Art and Science.

If I had the time, I would now, after forty-eight years of Osteopathy, reread all of Still and Sutherland and write a whole book on the Osteopathic Truths surrounding the Immune System. Why?

Because these Principles work so well in a variety of illnesses and support the functional reserve in the patient as a Wholeness ... the goal of healing.

To know Osteopathy, one must Live it in Practice ... this is the proving ground ... it is not a theory but an Art based in Oral Tradition.

Today there are theories upon theories about healing ... none ... absolutely none are better than what Osteopathy can offer in skilled and dedicated hands ... none!

If we dig deeper into the Basic Truths given to us by Still and Sutherland (without modification or turning these truths into techniques) ... it will lead to uncanny clinical results and great discoveries in yourself.

It will most definitely improve your Immune Function ... because the false images and ideas you have will fall away, leaving your own Health exposed "to be sensed as Yourself," a sensation that will heal your mind and soma of desire for any other source of knowing or healing.

The Health is at the Core of the Immune System.

Today the Science of Immunology is at the doorstep of ideas Still promoted one hundred years ago. The teaching in Medical Education about the Immune System is weak and pharmacologically oriented.

If you wish to study the Immune System you must reread Still, Sutherland .... and find books on the Immune System written about its Normal Activity ... not about how to treat diseases ... I recommend *The Neuro-Immune-Endocrine Connection* by Carl Cotman et al., published by Raven Press, 1987.

The goal of treatment is not to support the rationale of science as an end in itself but to bring the Health into the foreground ... centered in the Original Blueprint created as an Embryo.

The Science of Immunology calls this Original Blueprint the Self.

What Is This Self?

The Self is a Scientific term used in Immunology that means the Mind that Creates all the Systems of the Organism ... the Mind that never misses a perfect intersect in time and space, the Mind behind the building of all systems and their internal communication as a Singularity ...

Still called this Self the Health, the Wholeness of Mind, Matter, and Motion ... the Perfect that is Eternal in Us ... it is the infrastructure of the Immune System ...

The Self That Exists Before the Immune System Is Generated

As immunologists search for the location of this Self, they come up empty ... it is there, but their tools cannot find its location.

Where Is This Self Located?

The Place where Self Lives is in the Whole. It suffuses but has no location on an anatomical plane.

Dr. Still could hear it, smell it, see it, taste it, and touch the Touch that touched him. He knew this wholeness and referred to it as the Health.

How Did He Do This?

He was a Listener, an Observer, not a manipulator of Natural Law... Wholeness for him was a Reality that he could exchange with ... his Science was well ahead of the average clinical mind of today.

Wholeness as an experience is not centered in or from the Individual... the Self at the core of Wholeness senses a Oneness that has a distinct Intended motion. This will be our main exploration in Phase Eight.

As a healing force, the Self's purpose is to bring all the parts away from their bias into a Singularity ... this resynchronization occurs during Neutral.

The Immune System, as I said earlier, begins as a Wholeness known as the Self, which creates the Immune System as an Organ wherein the recognition of non-self requires the development of another self , different from the Self.

This new self is called self with a small s... this self can recognize "non-self" and make responses that create such things as antibodies, fever, and hormonal changes, which protect the individual from the "outside influence" that is seen as a threat.

Remember that Self can heal also, but a dramatic loss of self-interest is required before the transmutation of outside influences can occur. The genetics tend to promote little "self" formation in their own image.

As the self-image comes into the perceptual system, one begins to see other people more intensely as "non-self ." We outgrow our own well-being.

Perception Is an Immune Function.

When I first read about this, I thought "What?" ... As I read on, I began to understand it more easily. I adjusted my image of the Immune System to include Perception as the Senses operating from the Health and Perception with a small *p* as being connected to seeing others as separate from oneness!! ... that is, seeing others as less than or more than oneself ... some interesting insight came forth.

What does it mean to our well-being that Perception is an Immune Function? ... does how we see ourselves and others affect our well-being?

What does it mean that Autistic phenomena are primarily perceptual dysfunctions? ...

Perception is the orientation of the awareness; its fulcrum should be in the third ventricle and in relationship to Zone D (minimum). The centering of the awareness is a developmental process occurring around the third ventricle as part of Immune System dynamics ... (see The Neuro-Immune-Endocrine Connection).

The Perception resides in Self as an Embryo and stays there until the familial-social, environmental, and genetic influences (first six weeks) create another self, in whom the awareness is moved to a location of seeing non-self more as "not me" than as "me." With this change, the meaning of Love changes to something beneficial for me rather than the Whole of Life (which disappears from the awareness).

What effect does how someone sees you have on your sense of well-being?

If someone, or a Higher Presence, touches your Self as "you" ... what happens to your reserve ... to your capacity to heal ... to your sense of being Loved?

What if your little "self" is seen as you, by yourself or others? ... how do you feel?

What role does self-image play in Healing?

What role do others' expectations play in the creating of your self-image and non-self criteria? These elemental Perceptions are the role of environment in the false movement of "self" as Self... in a way that removes the Perception of self.

Let's Discuss Autoimmune Disease

The Self develops an Immune System that isolates "self" from "non-self" (designed to reject non-self by a variety of defenses) ... but what happens when self is seen as non-self ... when the self becomes a stranger, is seen as an antagonist, as a non-self?

One becomes "allergic to oneself," i.e., autoimmune disease ... conditions like Lupus and Rheumatoid Arthritis surface.

The worst case I have ever seen was in an eight-year-old redheaded quite intelligent and youthfully proud child.

He had come for well child treatments over the span of his childhood and was very much in control of his parents ...

Hepatitis Vaccine was given at the prompting of the pediatrician ... within hours the child had full-blown severe Juvenile Rheumatoid Arthritis ... the pediatrician saw no connection between the vaccination and the onset of the Autoimmune Disease ...

The child was brought to me for treatment ... his joints were awful! The treatment took two months and four sessions ... the Principles used are the ones we will do today with the "Bird" ... this was not an easy case to treat and the level of precision was challenging for me, but the outcome was a full recovery.

The Pediatrician talked the mother into a second injection of the Hepatitis vaccine...

The Arthritis immediately reappeared and was more severe and imbedded in his system than the first time ...

No response to treatment was forthcoming ... sadly, he never recovered...

His mother was angry and began to research the Hepatitis Vaccine. Being a lawyer, she was persistent in finding that Autoimmune problems were suspect during the production research of the Vaccine ... we lost contact after this.

Vaccinations can be costly. They are focused upon tricking the Immune system, which sometimes gets confused and turns on itself ...

The Immune System is so subtle and refined that it can only function well when there is the least possible "synaptic noise" in the central nervous system ... the need for relative Silence to make accurate discernment and respond appropriately is very necessary and often overlooked in our thinking.

In Autoimmune Dysfunction there is mass confusion in the synapses, an overload that results in an "identity crisis," which results in "self-rejection" ... then the self is seen as non-self.

In the above case, the child was excessively self- centered and very controlling of the parents, treating them as if they were stupid ... all this was obvious in visits prior to the vaccine reaction.

In Osteopathy, getting to the Cause is not always a simple Allopathic exercise ... in this case the child's sense of self was distorted and created a definite perceptual lesion that stressed the Immune Function ... the treatment never altered this basic problem because the parents were identified with the child being "superior" ... this sounds complex, but seen in the light of how the Immune System was experiencing the child, one could conclude that there was a lot of "noise" in the system and a definite perceptual lesion that was costly.

"Your Skill Is Proportionate to Your Understanding of Normal." (A. T. Still)

Not Disease!

If the Normal Immune System cannot think straight when there is too much synaptic noise, how then can we create quiet in the central nervous system so that the Immune System can return to its normal level of precision and discernment ... how can we help it REST?

Neutral

Neutral brings the movements of inhalation and exhalation to a balance point where the in and out of inhalation comes to the Stillness of its pivotal power ... this is a basis of the Osteopathic Principles we use in treatment ... Why?

Because Neutral is homeostatic. It is where the Organism reorients itself to the SELF... This is accomplished by Indwelling Therapeutic forces generated by Primary and Thoracic Respiration that pass into the Neutral Field and breath into it the Original Blueprint of the System.

Notice that we do not give the treatment but set the conditions for it to happen innately... this is basic... what we can do is help the Neutral emerge. We know this from prior Phases and other teaching, but ... to access the Immune System, the Neutral must reach a depth beyond rates, and into a Dynamic Stillness. This will be clear from the practical.

De-facilitation of synaptic noise in the Wholeness occurs as the Neutral emerges into the Dynamic Stillness, but at lower levels of Neutral the Immune System will not treat directly.

Facilitation, on the other hand, is the beginning of disease.

Synaptic noise pollutes the faculty of discernment and

weakens the Immune response … if facilitation goes to the core of the brainstem, then the reciprocal tension potency lesions in the third ventricle.

Why do we not remember the sensation of the real Health of the Self; how come we have forgotten …?

Loss of the Memory of the Health in the Soma develops from environmental and genetic influences as well as the structure of education.

The idea of being self-centering and independent is appealing to the pride, and so we involute in Memory. When we center events on the memory, the memory is of our lifetime, not the Movement of Life as a Whole.

Ultimately, we lose our discernment of Zone D and its Landscape. As we do so, we lose our direct interface with Nature, killing a large amount of innate gratitude that creates well-being … this leaves us grieving … unsettled. Nothing will ever fill this emptiness until the Memory returns … and our senses reawaken to the Presence itself.

As we practice listening with our hands rather than doing, doing, doing, and imposing ideas on the patient, we sometimes have a sense of being seen, or of being inside a Greater Reality … this is the first step in the recovery of Real Memory.

The sense of self begins to move from isolation and false self to being a part of a bigger picture … then we start to remember the sense of Self … something that does not need "non-self" … there is no need to reject or eliminate anyone or anything as a lesion. One sees but without a sense of other as "not me."

As we learn to reverse our sensorium and to listen for motion rather than stimulate motion … we begin to "hear" things we never heard before, and yet these new things seem to bring a sense of relief to the operator … our Memory unlocks slowly.

When we look for something we never saw before rather than our old format, and remain Still and Unmoved by temptations … we will then see the motion of the Long-Tide (long ago forgotten) and its pivotal essence in the Dynamic Stillness of the Sea Around Us.

Overview

The Immune System needs a Neutral, a Rest, a Pause from the frantic life imposed by our needs ... in the Rest, there comes a direct interchange with the Self ... but ... only if the Neutral is of sufficient depth—a depth of Silence and Stillness that lets the Immune System hear the Self, which then creates a Dynamic Interchange of form, chemistry, and synchronization recentering perception.

We will work in Phases Five and Six to better understand these sensations and listen to the language that speaks from the Self ... We will discuss more about the Immune System and Autism, a perceptual lesion in the Immune System.

Fever and the Immune System

Fever is immune fire ... it is electromagnetic in its actions ... it flows from the center (third ventricle) to the periphery (neurotrophic flow) into the lymphatic, where it discharges electricity into the fluid directly ... As the fire hits the passing white blood cells, it ignites an immune response that causes the cells to increase their antibody production by thousands of times. These antibodies then confront "non-self" ...

Still knew this ... his senses listened and he saw a great deal ... he knew fever was electrical ... he knew that the fire could only work if the Ignition of the Engine of Life was able to "fire" adequately.

The Engine of Life has its Ignition in the heart of the Bird, the third ventricle ... All this was "seen" before the Immunologists formulated their models ... now let's go back to the discussion about fever ...

In your bloodstream are observers that recognize "self" ... they are complex proteins called pyrogens ... when a "foreigner" enters the house, these pyrogens run off to the third ventricle ... they pass through the lamina terminalis, which, as part of the blood-brain barrier, allows the pyrogens to pass into the cerebrospinal fluid of the third ventricle ... think about the precision and Intelligence here ...

Once these pyrogens arrive in the third ventricle, they communicate the need for Fire (fever). If the third ventricle is healthy, the Ignition fires and makes fever.

The fever must get to the peripheral lymphatics to accomplish an adequate antibody response ... neurotrophic flow begins (if the third ventricle is able to perform normally) from the center to the periphery. The nerves channel this fire to the lymphatics, where, as we said before, the white blood cells are suffused with the fire and create a multitude of antibodies that impair the growth of the "Foreigner" (non-self).

Here is a system that boggles the imagination almost to the point of Awe.

Still was very clear; his thinking was always to support the immune response and the flow of the lymphatics ... Sutherland, in "The Tour of the Minnow," describes the Dynamics that Still saw.

Today Science is just coming to realize that inflammation is the source of stasis that causes many conditions, like coronary artery disease, arthritis, et al. ... the role of stasis and inflammation is connected to the motion of fire ignition and the third ventricle as a continuum in the Whole motion of Primary Respiration and its role in Immune Function.

Remember, the Potency of the Spark of Life Ignites the fire (potency with a little p) ... this is a key movement in the Immune System. The following motions are necessary for Immune Function:

Mind, the Divine Mystery

The Movement of the Breath of Life

The Spark of Creation ... Fire

Ignition

The Motion of Primary Respiration in the Individual

The Self (Health)

fire (little f)

The self/non-self interface

Instinct ... the indwelling Observer supporting Self

The accurate discernment of non-self

The Form and Function of the Neural Tube (Matter Moving)

The creation of potency (fire)

Direct trophic transmutation

Neurotrophic flow and discharge

Alignment of the awareness with the Horizon

Communication in a Sea of Quiet

The dependency of the Immune System on Self as the Overseeing Mind for the Immune System can be felt when Neutral maturates to the level of the Dynamic Stillness.

The terminology at the beginning of this commentary has specific meaning; each word has a function that one sees directly ... These are not just theory, but a physiological reality hidden from most of the Sciences, but not from the "listening still senses" that we are given for seeing ... Majesty in Motion.

CLINICAL APPLICATIONS

In acute febrile illness, like upper respiratory infections, the flu, et cetera, we know that the movement of the fever from the center of the third ventricle to the periphery is essential to limiting the disease.

If you check the head and the extremities, they both should be feverish.

Often what we see is that the head is extremely hot, the eyes glassy, the patient listless, and the extremities cool ... this means that the central febrile response has started but the neurotrophic flow is stalled so that the peripheral antibody response is minimal ... this means, of course, that this illness could become quite serious ... Osteopathic treatment based on our understanding of the Immune System could be very helpful in decreasing the morbidity of the illness.

The work we do with the Bird today will be a foundation for treating these cases successfully ... Remember, Still's reputation was made from his success in treating influenza, not structural dysfunctions.

The treatment will change the illness overnight, in most cases avoiding the use of medications or remedies.

In local inflammations with low fever, like when infants are cutting teeth, we use slightly different principles. The fever is in the third ventricle and the Anterior Cranium. Local treatment using the Stillness in the inflammatory movement itself will serve to help remove the inflammation and swelling, making the child less distressed. In this example, if the fever does not move to the Anterior Cranium, then the same treatment as we are doing today with the "Bird" will help.

Vaccines are notorious for "mixing up the Immune Clarity" … this requires a reorganization of the motion and orientation of the reciprocal tension potency, the third ventricle, the tissue motion present in the Neural tube, and the Ignition. We will cover this in later Phases, as we have only so much time.

THE OTHER PAIR OF HANDS

The presence of the "other pair of hands" was introduced to the profession in 1991 at a Sutherland Cranial Teaching Foundation conference. Many of the elders were interviewed to see if this "event" should be included in Osteopathic terminology. A few elders were aware of the "other pair of hands," but no one wanted to speak openly about it for fear of negative feedback. This fear has been an issue with Osteopathy in the Cranial Field as long as I have been an Osteopath.

I decided to speak and write about it because, if twenty or thirty people have witnessed it (without speaking with each other beforehand), then by definition it is Science. Also, if we as teachers deny what we experience, we limit everyone's progress. The task is to find what is common to many and teach that, not personal "gifts." Today, many people have confirmed that at times "the other pair of hands" appears and demonstrates treatment and teaching.

The Following Approach Works Well for Engaging This Help.

First, we must really need help. We must have reached the limit of our skill and been humbled by that limit.

Next, sense around the edge of the skin.

Sense for An Other Pair of Hands somewhere on that surface.

The rest is self-evident.

In the Treatment of Children, the Other Pair of Hands Appears Inside a Golden Fluid

CONCENTRATION

All of the Great Osteopaths were interested in the interface between "little mind" and Mind.

They all had incredible focus, intention, dedication, and attention, and could "see" things that the little mind could not see.

All of my teachers had Faith in a Greater Mind and searched for greater purity in themselves.

Our attention is our greatest gift, but, untrained, it will be moved away from the means toward an end, through the distractive nature of our ego, or "little mind."

We are steadfast in our belief in Neutral as a receptacle for the Indwelling Healing Forces to pour themselves into us, creating unexpected and meaningful outcomes in treatment. Neutral is a means, not and end. The end is accomplished not by us but by the Tide.

When the Tide has centered you, and the veil is lifted and you may see the Tide's intention, and also a lesion ... here is where you Concentrate ... Concentrate on the Presence of the Tide, its concerns, its power ... not yours, or your analysis of your relationship with the lesion ... Concentrate on the Tide and its Intention.

This Principle, set by Still and passed to us from the Elders, is now yours to nurture and to study ... and to assimilate ... then you can teach others when they are mature enough to know the difference between a technique and a "way of being."

Dedication to where you put your attention and when, and what you Concentrate your attention toward, is who you are and what degree of the Health you will experience.

Thank You

I have learned from the writings of Dr. Still, Dr. Sutherland, and many embryologists; from the oral teaching of many mentors including Ruby Day, Anne Wales, and Rollin Becker; from conversations with Bill Johnson and Alan Becker; and from the comments of my follow travelers in courses and study groups ... thousands of moments of help.

My goal, which came from the Tide, was to download everything I received from my teachers, so that the Beauty of what Osteopathy is can be remembered ...

Thank you.

BIODYNAMICS OF OSTEOPATHY BOOK SERIES

This book is one of a series of twelve *Biodynamics of Osteopathy* books. It is recommended that you read the whole series in order, as each book builds on the understanding from prior books. It is also recommended that you seek experienced teachers and mentors to help you experience the full depth of the information given.

The full series is as follows:

Phase One is about involuntary motion, which is motion present in the whole and in the lesion. We learn to synchronize with the breathing of Primary Respiration before we approach any treatment. This synchronization is the key to working with stable rates and not irritating the system. The principle of synchronizing with a healthy aspect of the patient suffuses the whole teaching program. This synchronization shifts our awareness to a different level of receptivity, which allows us to see Primary Respiration rather than the lesion field, and this eventually leads us to an understanding of the intention of Primary Respiration.

Phase Two is about communication with the natural laws of healing that surround activity at 2 to 3 cycles per minute. We synchronize with the breathing of Primary Respiration and also add the skill of sensing the fulcrum, the Stillness through which the breathing creates form and function. It is a different kind of synchronization from that in Phase One, shifting our awareness more deeply. As this occurs, the treatment automatically expresses itself. The end point of treatment, when compared with Phase One, reveals several differences. We find this kind of synchronization works exclusively with the fluid body and the outcome of treatment is more complete than when working with tissue alone.

Phase Three is centered around the activities of the Long Tide (100 second cycle). We explore an indwelling therapeutic force already present in the lesion field. We learn that the dural system is not made-up of three sickles but rather a series of folds in a sac, arising during growth and development. We see the relationship between the upper and lower dural sacs, awakening us to the independence of two separate tentorium cerebelli. We discover that zone D, the horizon, and the Wire (along which the Long Tide moves during its intended therapeutic course) are all linked as natural laws pertaining to this level of Primary Respiration.

Phase Four focuses on the Midline, a place where the spatial relationships are expressed as a whole. It synchronizes and centers us in such a way that we become aware of Zone D and the Dynamic Stillness. The Third Level Stillness in Phase Four is different from the Stillness in the other Phases – we are centered by the Stillness at the center of creation. Our intention is replaced by the intention of the Tide which can facilitate our spiritual path.

Phase Five is about *the face*. As we approach the face, we use all of the principles that we have learned in Phase One, Two, Three, and Four. We work with automatic shifting and notice differences from how the face is viewed by older models within Osteopathy in the Cranial Field. As we synchronize with the therapeutic presence of the Long Tide we see what we can learn about the face from that landscape. We also work with Seams, Dynamic Stillness, and Ignition.

Phase Six is a continuation of our journey into the Wholeness that generates life and delivers therapeutic forces that transmute lesions once Neutral is expressed. It is a mixture of activities centered around the outside presence of Primary Respiration as something that is a non-biological force and that has a persona. We will also continue to explore seams and then move on to the extremities, first in the embryological terms and then as Sutherland taught them in his work called PowerPoints. Phase 6 is a time to build your understanding of the Tide and refine your skills.

Phase Seven highlights the Health. Dr. Still's famous comment "Find the Health; anyone can find disease," has plagued many minds over the last century. We come to the clear vision of several indwelling aspects of the Health: Love ... liquid light ... and a diamond matrix. A approach to the terminally ill and dying patient is addressed. In the somatic sensation of the Tide passing through the House Under the Sea, our awareness is transmuted by the Health. The lesion is seen as a precognitive act of the Health. Thoracic Respiration, Primary Respiration, and Ignition are as One. The landscape is vast ... and the principles of healing are even more substantial than we have previously experienced..

Phase Eight is a deeper exploration of seams, balanced rhythmic interchange, and the Flame of Intention as a therapeutic modality. Phase Eight is the culmination of our awareness of Wholeness, and ultimately brings us to the Divine Presence, Unconditional Love and Oneness. The living Tide dominates the awareness while forms move to the background. One feels the Breath of Creation in oneself as the Center of Wholeness. One feels the Unfoldment of oneself as one is Created. Our consciousness is a gift; we do not own it and if we try to control it we lose Wholeness.

Phase Nine is when we are able to fully evaluate and treat the Central Nervous System and the Eye. We also address Fire and the therapeutic modality of the Shakedown. True action is moved from Love and makes our perception exist. This Love is self-emptying and by its nature allows us to Serve as part of the Perfect. Perception can be used to Serve something other than ourselves. We have attempted to enter this balance point between the Perfect and the Disease ... it is a point where the whole of everything is suspended by Love as it works to incarnate the Complete. In the balance point of everything is The Intention of the Tide following the movement of the distortion back to a True relationship with the Blueprint of Life.

Pediatrics One explores how children grow as a whole, not in parts as we sometimes believe. Children live in the Direction of Ease of motion present in their fluid metabolic fields, otherwise they get uncomfortable and require assistance. Does your treatment directly support the whole, or does it assume to support the whole? We realize children are not adults and cannot be treated as adults are. We approach the therapeutic modality of the "Meeting Place", prenatal and postnatal periods, the treatment of the pelvis during pregnancy, fetal malposition and labor.

Pediatrics Two is where we deepen in the perceptive awareness necessary to approach the treatment of children. We deepen in our appreciation of Wholeness, the three levels of Stillness and the "Meeting Place". We approach "Desert Neutral", where therapeutics pass into the neutral substance, and a mystery unfolds as the breath of Divine love cascades as a therapeutic force across a night desert landscape, filling and leaving behind no visible effects. We further address treatment of the pelvis and the uterus during pregnancy. We explore thoracic and Primary Respiration in children, and the Family Circle.

Pediatrics Three is where we continue to study the therapeutic Flow of Attention. We deepen in Third Level Stillness and the Meeting Place. The Meeting Place is easily misinterpreted … our observer must be so still and neutral that the process can be seen as it happens. The central nervous system in the child can be finally approached for evaluation and treatment. We explore teething and also the "locked up head". We use the therapeutic modality of the Flame of Intention, and its connection to the Breath of Life. Everything is transparent to the Breath of Life.

ABOUT THE AUTHOR

James Jealous, D.O. (1943–2021), was an osteopathic physician, teacher, and writer. His life's work was founding and developing **Biodynamics of Osteopathy**, a unique methodology he established within the field of osteopathy, following the lineage of Dr. A.T. Still and Dr. W.G. Sutherland.

He was born in Saco, Maine, and since his father was an osteopathic physician, he was around osteopathy from an early age. He studied at Kirksville College of Osteopathic Medicine in Missouri (now the A.T. Still University of Health Sciences), graduating in 1970. He then set up practice in rural Maine as an osteopathic primary care physician.

Over time, Dr. Jealous saw parallels between the work of embryologist Dr. Erich Blechschmidt and that of osteopathic physician Dr. William Garner Sutherland. This inspiration led him to create his own body of work. In the early 1990s, he began teaching "A Biodynamic View of Osteopathy in the Cranial Field," which, as he developed his specific methodology, was refined to "Biodynamics of Osteopathy."

A deeply spiritual person, he felt most at home in the natural world and was an avid fisherman and hiker.

For more information, please visit:
https://BiodynamicsOfOsteopathy.com

There is a wind passing through …
it is the motion of creation,
the eternal motion of Divine love.